If Diets Don't Work, What Does?

A Doable, Enjoyable Guide to Living the Life You Want

Danielle Dinkelman, NBC-HWC
National Board Certified Health & Wellness Coach

Editorial work by Michele Preisendorf

Cover design by Mahmud Didar

Photography by Heather Clark

Interior print design and layout by Rachel Bostwick

Ebook design and layout by Rachel Bostwick

ISBN: 9798721077487

Praise for If Diets Don't Work, What Does

"A great combination of easy to understand information and practical tips! The questions at the end of the chapters allow each reader to reflect on their own journey and personalize their experience with the material."

-Suzanna Cooper, Chief Learning Officer at Catalyst Coaching Institute

"Danielle has a real gift for finding the right tools to overcome every obstacle to your success for health and well-being."

-Jane Birch, PhD, Author of *Discovering the Word of Wisdom: Surprising Insights from a Whole Food, Plant-based Perspective*

"Danielle's book is a spark of hope to anyone seeking to make positive changes in life. Her approach is strongly based in science while still being accessible."

-Mallory Barrick, cookbook developer and founder of sonderity.com

"Danielle's voice is like a knowledgeable and intuitive friend who nurtures and believes in the reader's ability to create lasting lifestyle change. This book is full of useful, science backed, tools and opportunities to reflect and gain important insights along the journey to a healthier life."

-Yvette Morton Ed.S, MA, NBC-HWC, Student Success & Wellbeing Coach

"Danielle's book shares the refreshing truth that health is not about beating ourselves into good habits, but loving our bodies and believing in ourselves so we naturally achieve our best self. This book feels like a personal cheerleader in your hand—an empowering friend we all need!"

-Faith Ralphs, plant-based recipe developer and founder of FaithfulPlateful.com

"A must read if you have been a chronic dieter your whole life, and you are tired and ready to stop the madness. Danielle's beautiful approach helps you stop the diet mentality and begin the process to come home to yourself and start your journey to true health."

-Tricia Braunersrither, host of *Wisdom with Trish* Podcast

For my mother, Tracy—the woman who taught me to be myself and live my joy.

Contents

Introduction

There's Got to Be Another Way

Diets suck. There, I said it. You know it's true.

But if diets don't work, what does? I have seen many women and men in my life try to leave dieting behind and try to just focus on a healthy lifestyle, only to struggle and give up. So what does it take to be successful in the lifestyle approach to health?

This is the question I asked myself when I started out as a health coach. I knew I wanted to help people, but I saw much awry in the wellness world. People were confused by conflicting information, overwhelmed by the task of change, and frustrated by recurring failure. What do people need to be successful in creating the lives they want?

This book is a summation of the discoveries I have made on how we can reclaim and maintain our health with a lifestyle approach. My perspective has been marvelously shaped by positive psychology; wellness-coaching techniques; the whole-food, plant-based movement; behavior-change science, spirituality; mindfulness; and more.

This book gives you a philosophy you can live by and a process you can use to make your efforts in healthy living as effective, enjoyable, and realistic as possible.

As you read each chapter and apply what you learn, you can create a personalized approach to your health journey. There are journal prompts at the end of each chapter to help you do this. You'll also have access to bonus materials, including videos, templates, and other resources, to help you go deeper and take action.

I am so excited for you to be able to make sustainable changes. You will know how to make your journey doable and enjoyable. You will learn how to set yourself up for success. Doesn't that sound better than the alternative? You will never have to diet again. You can absolutely reclaim your health with lifestyle, one step at a time.

The Lay of the Land

This book consists of twelve short chapters. I could write five times this much on the subject, but it is more important that my message is clear, concise, and practical. What good would it be otherwise?

As you read this book, you'll learn everything you need to know about getting started on your way to a healthy, sustainable lifestyle. It will be uniquely yours. I will give you the roadmap, but you must take the journey.

First, we'll uncover the problems with dieting. More than just the ridiculous, overly restrictive recommendations of the typical fad diet, you will come to see the REAL problem with diets: unsustainable change.

Next, I'll invite you to picture the life you want. If you could create it from scratch, what would it be like? What do you want in health and life? Of course, we must then explore possible excuses, or the "Yeah, buts," that will inevitably show up to stop you. But don't worry—it's part of the process. I will help you face your demons head-on. Only then can you do the mental work it will take to make this next stage of your health journey different and better than ever.

Once you're grounded in your purpose and vision for your life and health, you will learn how to take an effective lifestyle approach to wellness. You will learn the basics of behavior-change science that have revolutionized the health journey of each and every one of my clients. (Turns out science knows how to make lasting change; most of us out in the real world just haven't heard about it yet.)

With your feet firmly planted in sustainable change strategies, then and only then can we talk about the five aspects of healthy living. You'll explore the powerful effects of prioritizing sleep, upgrading nutrition, finding enjoyable exercise, managing stress with self-care, and remodeling your mindset. Each chapter invites you to consider what YOUR next best step could be.

Finally, we sum it all up by remembering why we began in the first place. You want to feel your best so you can give your all. You deserve to feel better, and you believe feeling better is possible. It is—as long as you don't quit.

At the end of each chapter, there are introspective exercises I call "Journal Prompts." These are the type of questions and exercises I use with clients in my coaching programs. If you truly wish to get the most out of this book, don't skip these exercises. The journal prompts will help you take what you read and apply it. There are no right or wrong answers. Only your answers.

What's in it for You

So, are you ready? Are you excited? Nervous? Hesitant? Ready to slam this book shut and say "Never mind"? It's okay. I get it. You've probably been burned by programs and promises before. I want you to know that all of my clients feel uneasy at the beginning. So let me tell you what this book is and what it is not.

This book is not a one-size-fits-all *program*. It's a philosophy and a process.

This book is not a silver bullet. There is not one thing alone that will solve all your frustrations. This book is designed to be taken as a whole and applied as you are ready, willing, and able.

This book is not a one-off solution. One-and-done will not do. The things you learn here need to sink in deep, so reading it again and again is advised. Think of it as your trusty companion on a long, beautiful journey.

This book is not a magic pill. There are no guarantees. You will find guidance and guidelines, but the definitive answers you are looking for are not on these pages—they are in your mind and gut. Follow your intuition as you read, and you will not go wrong.

So why should you keep reading? What can you really expect to gain from something that claims to be so new and so different from all the rest?

I'll tell you.

I wrote this book so you could learn how to *feel your best so you can give your all*. Here's how:

- By reading this book, you'll see how to practice SUSTAINABLE change.

- You'll gain inspiration from others who have chosen the lifestyle approach to health.

- You'll see how to make YOUR journey doable *and* enjoyable.

- You will learn the process of positive change.

- You will learn what it takes to make lifestyle change work for you.

- You will learn how to not quit.

- You will get crystal clear on the ideal aspects of healthy living: what to stop and what to start doing (when you're good and ready).

- You will feel empowered as you learn simple strategies for healthy living.

- You will see how you can prioritize your health without letting people down.
- You will learn about the power of choosing self-compassion in the face of setbacks.
- You will start to rebuild self-trust and restore body trust.
- You will weed out the lies and myths diet culture has planted in your brain (knowingly or unknowingly).

And my favorite of them all:

You will learn how to start living vibrantly NOW—one layer, one step at a time. No more "I'll be happy when." You get to choose happiness now, regardless of your results.

I am so glad you are here. I am so glad you are choosing a better way. Be brave. Be gentle. Be at peace, and let's begin.

1

If Diets Don't Work, What Does?

MY CLIENT'S DOCTOR SAT HER DOWN to give her the talk about her weight. He explained the health risks she faced. He used the word obese three times, which felt like a slap in the face that stung repeatedly. Then he proceeded to promote the "perfect solution" for her. "Ideal protein," he said. "It's wonderful because you lose weight fast and you don't even need to exercise." My client was flabbergasted. Why would a doctor be telling her to biohack her way to weight loss? It seemed so wrong.

Dieting seems to be a given in modern life. Everywhere you look, there's a new pill or program that promises quick and exaggerated results. With so many testimonials and convincing before-and-after photos, it's easy to get sucked into the diet culture. It's alluring to think one of those paths contains all the answers to all your health problems and frustrations.

I believe that at our core, we all know getting healthy is about more than starting the next fad diet. It's time for a big-picture perspective on health and wellness. It's time every man, woman, and child knows what it takes to create health and maintain it. It's time that vibrant, healthy living be attainable for every one of us. What's more, it's high time getting healthy is enjoyable!

If you're like most of the women and men I've worked with, you've been there, done that with diets. You've tried everything! And although you can get your results with the best of them and shrink your body whenever you want, you're tired of yo-yo dieting. You're tired of having to muster enough grit and willpower to follow their extreme six-week regimen. You're exhausted. You just want to live your life! You've come to realize that fad diets are not focused on health. And even though you know you can jump on the next bandwagon and lose twenty to fifty pounds at will, you're not sure how that could ever be sustainable.

In this book, I'll walk you through what to do instead of dieting. I will teach you how to be successful with a lifestyle approach. I promise that as you let me guide you through this next stage of your journey, you will be able to take what I teach and apply it to your life in a way that is absolutely unique to you. You can create a healthy lifestyle you love and a healthy lifestyle that loves you back for years and years to come.

My Wake-Up Call

Health challenges suck, but they sure do have a way of getting our attention. At nineteen, as I was finishing up my freshman year of college, I was in a life-changing car accident. I walked away from the eighty-five-mile-per-hour freeway rollover with barely a scratch on the outside, but on the inside, my body was wrecked. For the next four years, I was plagued with chronic pain and excruciating headaches. With pain as my new normal, I got married, graduated college, and had my first child. From the outside looking in, my life seemed pretty good. Living it, though, was hellish. I wasn't myself. The pain in my neck and shoulders persisted in spite of physical, chiropractic, and massage therapies. Finally, after four years of frustration and hopelessness, I met with a health professional who empowered me to do something about my situation.

After listening to my complaints, she said, "What are you doing to take care of your body after you leave my office?" A little embarrassed, I realized I really had nothing to say. I ate a junk-food diet, and I had no exercise routine to speak of. I was just a frustrated, pain-stricken mess. That's when we made a plan. I started experimenting with yoga in an effort to keep my poor damaged muscles lengthened and happy in between massage appointments. Soon, I added running (which my high school track-team friends would be shocked to know—I always thought they were nuts). And you know what? It worked! As I made a daily and weekly practice of yoga and worked up from walking to jogging to running, my body finally started to find a new normal that did not include disrupting my life with constant aches and pains.

Isn't it funny how life has its own plan for us? I would never have thought I'd be someone who loved yoga and running. Sooner or later, life will make you care about your health and wellness.

As my health improved, the rest of my life did too. When I was in pain, I was not the mother I wanted to be. I was short-tempered and irritable. My poor two-year-old was a trooper for putting up with me. What a miracle it was that implementing simple routines helped the pain subside to where I finally felt better and could be the happy, smiling mother I wanted to be. Health is not just physical—it's mental and emotional. It's all connected. When you start to pay attention and shift things in one area, it affects the others.

The same goes for health in relation to our life's purpose, don't you think? When we are not well, we can't fully live out our purpose. When I was not well, I was not the mother I wanted to be—or the wife, daughter, or friend, for that matter!

Can you relate? How are health challenges holding you back?

Why You? Why Now?

What about you? What's your story? If you were a new coaching client, I would want to hear all about it: where you've been up to this point, what obstacles you've faced, what you've tried to do about it, and how it's all gone so far. I would want to know about your wake-up call to health. What finally made you say "Enough is enough"? What was your wake-up call to wellness?

If now is the time to take charge of your health, I would like to know why. Why do you want to feel better? What are you not able to do right now that you wish you could? How is ill health holding you back? (Remember, these questions and others will be in your journal prompts at the end of the chapter, so keep reading for now and take some time to pause at the end and write down your responses then.)

Let's face it, health is a means to an end—not an end unto itself. We don't want to get healthier just so we can pin a badge on our chest and say "Look at me, I'm healthy!" No. It's more than that. You want to feel better so you can show up as the person you want to be. Whether you're a parent, grandparent, executive or manager, or business owner, people depend on you. People are influenced and impacted by you. Who you are to others is part of your purpose on this planet. So answer this: What's your purpose? How could you better fulfill your purpose if you were the healthiest possible version of yourself?

The answer to that question is part of why you deserve to feel better. You deserve to feel better because the people in your life deserve the best you have to offer. But you know what? You just deserve to have some joy and satisfaction in your life too! Maybe there are things you've always wanted to do but couldn't because of your health.

I say "No more!" No more settling. No more feeling helpless. That's why you're reading this book! Deep down, you believe you deserve better, and you want to believe that better is possible.

I'm here to tell you that better IS possible. You CAN reclaim your health with the principles of healthy living I will guide you through in this book. What's more, I believe you can reclaim your health ON YOUR OWN TERMS. I don't want you to do this because you "should." I want you to do this because you want to! And I will show you how to **customize a version of healthy living that is enjoyable and doable for *you*.**

Your Healthy Lifestyle Game Plan

I have seen many women and men leave dieting behind and lean into a healthy lifestyle approach only to flounder, struggle, and ultimately give up. It's hard to abandon the promises and guarantees of dieting. The lifestyle approach works, but only if you have a game plan. Consider this book your playbook.

People who succeed in the lifestyle approach have their bases covered (to use another sports analogy). They know the WHY, HOW, and WHAT when it comes to change. It only works if you have all three. Having just one piece will not work. Those who fail may know WHY they want to change, and so they depend 100 percent on their own willpower and motivation but eventually peter out. Others focus solely on WHAT to change, like diet or exercise. The pitfall I most often see is a lack of knowledge regarding the five aspects of health and wellness. These people put all their eggs in one basket and expect it to solve all their health problems. And they are often disappointed.

Knowing HOW to change has proven to be very rare indeed. Anyone can force a *temporary* six-week change, but few understand how to make the lifestyle approach work and how to make it last. That is where behavior-change science and taking charge of habits is absolutely indispensable.

In the chapters that follow, my goal is to simply and clearly give you the essential tools to leverage your WHY, be intentional with HOW, and be complete in WHAT you do to turn your health around.

If you have struggled to leave dieting behind and find a way to make a healthy, lasting lifestyle change, I am so glad you are here. I am absolutely confident that the principles, tools, and strategies you will get from this book will help you be successful. This book contains much of what I work on with my health coaching clients, and I have seen my approach work again and again for them. It can work for you as well.

I know it is hard to believe that this next step will be different. I know you've been through a lot. I know your confidence may be floundering. So that's why, right now, I want you to make just one commitment to yourself. Simply commit to reading this entire book in the next thirty days.

If you'll stay with me to the end, I promise you will have clarity and confidence when it comes to reclaiming your health naturally and joyfully. Each chapter includes journal prompts you can use to personalize the things you're learning. **You can download the *Journal Prompts Workbook* at danielledinkelman.com/toolkit. If you complete these and send them to me when you're done reading, you will get a free forty-five-minute VIP coaching session with me.** I can't wait for you to learn everything you can from this book! I look forward to connecting with you when you're done and helping you plan your next steps in your health journey.

As you read, you may start to feel resistance, fear, shame, defeat, or hopelessness bubble up inside you. This is normal. It's a sign that the old you is freaking out about the unknown. When you start to feel these uncomfortable feelings or think defeating thoughts, promise me you will press on. Keep reading. Tell yourself you don't have to jump into DOING anything. All you need to do is read. Let the words of this book paint a new picture of possibilities for you. Just keep reading.

What This Book Is NOT

Now, I know you've probably been through a lot up to this point. If you're in the same boat as 95 percent of the clients I've worked with, you've been through the wringer on all things dieting and health. So you might be wondering, how is this book any different from all the other books and programs out there?

That's a fair question. Most health programs and diets (even really evidence-based ones) have too much of a one-size-fits-all approach. That can lead to feeling a whole lot of guilt and shame if you're not doing it "just right." Guilt is a pretty weak motivator. I'm here to help you find a new way forward. You need a lot less guilt and a little more grace.

Other health programs and diets try to tell you *exactly* what steps to take. I'm not here to do that. On the contrary, it's time to trust your intuition in your health journey. Because each human is so incredibly unique, we are much better off when we learn correct principles and then govern ourselves.

Furthermore, when you sign up for a health program or commit to a certain diet, you tend to give away your power. You put 100 percent of your trust in the program and just go through the motions. I'm more interested in helping you find your *own* way forward because if it's YOUR idea, you're much more likely to do it (and enjoy it)!

Human nature is a funny thing. I once saw a meme that said, "I was going to do that, and then you told me to." It makes me laugh every time because it is SO TRUE! We humans do not like being told what to do. So why do we keep signing up for diets and health programs that dictate every move we should make, and then get frustrated when we find ourselves "rebelling" and falling off the bandwagon?

Well, good news, my friend: there's no bandwagon here. I hesitate to even call this book a "program." If it is a program, it's "built to suit," for sure. So please, please remember: There is no such thing as one size fits all. When it all comes down to it, no one can do this for you. Only you know the best way forward. Please try to trust your intuition more. This journey is yours and yours alone.

Let's Tailor This to YOU

Your health journey is a lot like going on vacation. There are countless ways you can spend your time, but only you know what will make it most enjoyable and meaningful for you. Wouldn't it be awful to show up at your destination and the guide you hired forced you to see all the historic museums when all you wanted to see was the rain forest?

On the other hand, what if they were on the other side of the spectrum and asked you what you wanted to see that day but offered no recommendations or guidance on how to experience what was most important to you? Don't you agree that the best experience is somewhere in between? Wouldn't you like a guide who listened to your input *and* offered some recommendations but who ultimately let you make the final decision? Of course you would! Your health journey is no different.

The diets and rigid programs of the past are like that guide who dictates your every move. Going it alone on a "healthy lifestyle," though, is just as frustratingly fruitless as the pushover guide who leaves 100 percent of travel in a foreign land up to you. What you learn in this book will equip you with everything you need to find the best way forward in a manner that is both effective and personalized.

I am so committed to this idea of customizing my approach with each and every client that I wish every person had a health-and-wellness coach of their own. There is nothing more rewarding than helping another human being find their way forward. While I cannot completely coach you through a book (let's be honest, it's a bit of a one-sided conversation here), I can give you all the tools and strategies I give my clients.

I will also share bonus materials to help you get even more clarity on your next steps. Each tool is designed to help you self-coach and customize what you learn in this book. These videos and downloads are all available at danielledinkelman.com/toolkit.

So this is it. You embark now! Are you excited? Are you nervous? Are you skeptical? It's all okay. Remember, all you need to do for now is keep reading. I look forward to supporting you here in this book.

I know this book will help you be successful. My greatest hope for you is that you find this journey enjoyable. No more white-knuckling it. No more deprivation. No more beating yourself up when life happens. No more of that. Keep reading to discover how to go about this journey with ease and joy. I can hardly wait! Let's do this.

TOOLKIT:

- PDF—Journal Prompts Workbook

CHAPTER 1 JOURNAL PROMPTS

1. What attempts have you made at living a healthy lifestyle? What worked? What didn't?

2. What wake-up call to health have you had?

3. Why is now the time to take charge of your health?

4. How is your health holding you back from living the life you want?

5. If you could have it your way, what would your health journey include? What do you need for it to feel DOABLE? What do you need for it to feel ENJOYABLE?

2

The Problem with Diets

WHEN I WAS ABOUT TEN YEARS old, I remember overhearing some women talking about dieting. One of them said, "Yep. You know if I can pinch an inch, it's time to go back on a diet!" I remember going into the bathroom and lifting my shirt to see how my belly measured up. Could I pinch an inch? To my dismay, I could! I'd never thought of myself as overweight, but this was the first time I considered it.

Whether you've been on a hundred diets in your life or none, we have all been affected by diet culture. In fact, one survey showed that 75 percent of American women endorse unhealthy thoughts, feelings, or behaviors related to food or their bodies.[1] This is diet culture in action. It changes us. It changes our relationship with things in the world that should be neutral, if not benevolent. It changes how we see the body we live in and the fuel we feed it.

If you are going to be successful in turning your health around with a lifestyle approach, you must become aware of the ways diet culture is informing your perspective on "healthy" eating and health in general. Let's start with this myth: "Being thin makes you healthy." There is no silver bullet for health. Dieting is not the answer because it is not holistic enough. Dieting ignores the other aspects of health and wellness, namely exercise and stress management. What's more, fad diets, by nature, are not sustainable.

Dieting is old news. Its time is past. You are ready for a new and better way to reclaim your health! Just like history, we must understand our past so we can create a better future. So think of this chapter as a guided tour through the dusty halls of diet culture. I'll be your guide in this slightly troubling museum. This is where you will see clearly the old, antiquated way of changing our behavior and shrinking our bodies. As you see it for the oppressive, harmful, deceiving thing it is, you'll be all the more committed to leaving it behind forever. In the chapters to come, we'll explore a better way—a holistic, healthy way—to live the life you want. First, though, you will get to look diet culture in the face and tell it, "No, Mr. Diet, I am done with you."

Before we begin, let's be clear on how we are defining *diet*. *Diet* or *dieting* can mean different things to different people. Here is my definition for this book: *dieting is any extreme restriction or change in eating behavior that induces feelings of deprivation and is unsustainable.* When I say "diet," I am referring to fad diets—those that promise quick and dramatic results in a short amount of time. Even if done for good reasons, like for at-risk individuals who are legitimately overweight or obese and have any number of health problems, including diabetes or heart disease, a diet is still a diet in my book.

So what's the problem with diets? Well, for starters, they just don't work long-term. Ninety-five percent of dieters will regain the weight they lose in one to five years.[2] NINETY-FIVE PERCENT! That is a crime against humanity when you consider that 45 million Americans go on a diet each year.[3] I say no more. The next fad diet is NOT your solution. YOU are. You are capable of so much more than climbing on the diet roller coaster. Let's stop being duped by diet culture. It's time to pull back the curtain and see what's really going on with diets. We must expose why diets don't work so you will commit to leaving their lies behind once and for all.

You're Not a Racehorse

Have you ever seen the blinders they put on racehorses? They put even larger blinders on horses that pull wagons or carriages. Blinders prevent horses from looking anywhere but directly in front of them. Diets do this to you. Diets give you tunnel vision. Diets force you to look at one thing and one thing only: the number on the scale.

There is a big difference between "going on a diet" and simply making a healthy change in diet. You can call it lots of things: eating healthier, changing your way of eating, adopting a healthier lifestyle. Those are some of the word choices my clients and I prefer. Most of the women and men who come to me for health-and-wellness coaching want me to help them make a healthy diet change. We do this in an enjoyable and sustainable way based on the principles you'll learn in chapter 8. Again and again, though, I see well-meaning recovering dieters bring their old dieting mentality to their new healthy lifestyle, and it gets in their way.

About a year ago, I started working with a client who had adopted my eating program but was frustrated that she hadn't lost weight. She shared that she was doing all the right things nutritionally, which should have allowed her body to shed the excess weight, but it wasn't happening for her, and she felt like a failure. She was frustrated and confused, to say the least. In one of our coaching calls, I asked what other benefits she had noticed as a result of her healthier way of eating. She responded with a laundry list of changes! Less pain and inflammation in her joints, less fatigue, less brain fog, and more energy. She even said she felt light on her feet. What's more, she also noticed her relationship with food was changing and she was not falling into mindless eating anymore. It was clear that her body was responding to her healthy eating, just not in the way she wanted most. No weight loss. No satisfaction. That is diet culture talking.

So, I ask you, is the scale stealing your joy? Are you completely fixated on ONE outcome? If so, you're not alone. One of the biggest lies of diet culture is that the only thing that matters is our weight. To leave that faulty thinking behind, stop dismissing the results that matter. Commit now to celebrate every little way that your body will thank you for the healthy changes you make. Trust your body to get to the weight loss when it's ready.

As you step into a healthier way of eating, don't put all your eggs in one basket. Changing your eating alone is another form of tunnel vision diet culture promotes. If we truly want to become healthy, we need to be holistic in our approach and pay attention to ALL aspects of health and wellness, not just nutrition.

The Problem with Finish Lines

One of the biggest beefs I have with diets is that they have a beginning and an end. Diets have a finish line. If you're solely focused on one short-term outcome, like dropping fifty pounds, you will do whatever it takes to accomplish that. And then what? I'll tell you. You'll join ranks with the 95 percent who gain back every pound they lost.

Health is not a freaking sprint. You cannot white-knuckle your way into a healthy lifestyle. Finish lines (aka weight-loss goals) in diet culture teach us to sacrifice at all costs AND look forward to the light at the end of the tunnel, when the prize is yours and the torture is over. Again, I say "No more!" Don't chase the finish line; chase the lifestyle. This goes for those of you choosing healthy eating to reverse lifestyle disease as well. If we want true and lasting health, we need to go about creating it in a way that is perpetual as well as pleasing.

If you have ever gone to unsustainable lengths to reach an end result, you may have experienced something I call the rubber-band effect. When you stretch so far and work so hard you are using every ounce of willpower you can muster just to reach your goal, there will come a time when you cannot help but "snap back" to your starting point. Slap! Can you feel it? The stinging, red welt? That's what diet culture does. It gives big promises, requires too much, and then dumps you right back to where you started.

Even if you press forward, read this book in its entirety, and begin crafting your own healthy lifestyle, it will all be for nothing if you do not cleanse this "finish line" mentality from your programming. To take a lifestyle approach is to make a lifelong commitment. It means letting go of finish lines. It means loosening your grip on "results." It means focusing more on the journey and letting the outcomes take care of themselves. More on this later in chapters 5 and 6, but for now, open your eyes to the times the alluring finish-line mentality ruled your life. If you're willing to be done with dieting, you have to be done with finish lines. You cannot sprint to good health like you can sprint to weight loss. It's time to start playing the long game. I promise I will show you how to play that game in a way you won't hate.

Huge Effort for Short-Term Results

Next on our tour of old, inadequate, ineffective ways to change behavior and get healthier is the practice of putting forth huge effort for short-term results. This is closely related to the problem of finish lines but definitely deserves its own attention.

"Go big or go home" is one of the mantras of dieting. It is dangerous to believe that in order to get results, you have to make huge changes all at once. This flies in the face of behavior-change science. "Go big or go home" doesn't serve you. It sets you up for failure. In fact, huge effort often leads to huge burnout. After all, there's a reason they call it a "crash diet."

I have met many women and men in my coaching practice who tell me they have tried and failed and tried and failed so many times at changing to a healthier lifestyle. Many of the people I work with come to me because they know I am a plant-based-nutrition advocate. Again and again, I hear their stories of failure and frustration in trying to make that disciplined way of eating a new lifestyle for themselves. Every time, I have to teach them that going cold turkey or changing eating habits overnight is not realistic. You can't just flip a switch and expect things to be different. You have to work with your habits if you're going to change them, and that takes time.

Speaking of time, let's talk about before and after pictures. I know you want one. I know you want to shed your health problems and see yourself healthier and happier. I know you want it now. Again, the culture we live in perpetuates this desire. Social media and marketing messages are mostly well-meaning but can mess with our brains to where we believe we can transform ourselves as quickly and easily as a snapshot. Before and after photos don't show the time that has passed. They don't show the plateaus. They don't show the setbacks. They don't show the behaviors and habits that have changed along the way. They are a tiny, one-dimensional view of a life-changing process. I bet you care more about the process than you think. I bet you want the growth and personal development that will come as you do the work. If so, it's time to stop killing yourself for that before and after picture.

Like all the other doctrines of diet culture, it's tempting to make a big, flashy commitment to yourself, whether it's a commitment to a diet or healthy lifestyle change, and expect that to be enough. The persuasive, pervasive sludge of diet culture we all swim through every day of modern life makes us think that this is the way to make changes. It's not. I'll show you why in chapter 7, but for now, just promise me: no more white-knuckling it. There is a better way. Keep reading, and I'll show you.

All-or-Nothing Thinking

The next attraction on our tour of the old dieting way is probably something you thought was just part of you and not cultural conditioning. I have yet to meet a recovering dieter who did not suffer from the sickness of all-or-nothing thinking. While you think you are a perfectionist by nature, I would argue that it is more by nurture and by diet-culture brainwashing that many of us become perfectionists.

Perfectionism in dieting has taught you this mantra: "If I'm not miserable, it might not work." I'm here to tell you, you don't have to be perfect to get results. Perfectionism in dieting has taught you to buy in to "No pain, no gain." These are not truths; they are lies. Sure, you may have to follow fad diets to the letter to get the promised results, but we absolutely cannot continue applying dieting mentalities to healthy living. And so I'll say it again: you do not have to be perfect to get results with healthy living.

I have seen this diet-culture fallacy play out for many of my clients. Recently, I was on the phone with a woman whose story was wrought with perfectionism. It hurt me to hear her talk about how her perfectionism often led to a "shame spiral" whenever she "cheated" in her new way of eating. (Side note: Beware of diet-culture language! It's a sign you are still being brainwashed!) She told me she had learned all about healthier plant-based eating and wanted to do it 100 percent but was sad to say she probably only ate the way she wanted to 70 percent of the time. That's when I taught her about the pendulum effect.

The pendulum effect is when something isn't working over here on one side (say, 70 percent healthy eating) and we overreact! It's almost like overcorrecting your steering when you suddenly realize you are drifting into the other lane. You freak out and yank as hard as you can (swinging the pendulum over to 100 percent). Do you see how unhelpful and unnecessary this is? Just because 70 percent healthy eating isn't helping you feel better or lose weight, it does not mean you must jump all the way to 100 percent to get what you want!

While perfectionism won't serve you, mediocrity won't either. The most successful clients notice where they want to improve, take small but mighty steps forward, and steadily raise the bar. Bit by bit is the way to go. No overcorrecting. No pendulum swings. Just slow and steady progress.

I'll tell you right now, you do not have to eat perfectly, sleep perfectly, exercise perfectly, eliminate all stressors imaginable, or have a pristinely perfect mindset to get results from a healthy lifestyle. I could name multiple clients who have said, "I'm so relieved I don't have to be perfect to feel better." Every step in the direction of health will make a difference. Getting healthy is not about being perfect. It's about making progress. It's not so much about what you're doing or not doing; it's about moving and not standing still. As you continue reading, you will begin to remodel your understanding of how to make healthy changes based on behavior science, NOT on diet culture.

One Size Fits None

As we wrap up our final vignette of modern diet culture, it's time to expose the most insidious lie of all. Diet after diet, fad after fad has stood up in the public square and preached, "Here, this is your answer," "Just do exactly as I say and you can be thin and healthy like everyone else." It's tempting. You want to believe it. You want to believe they have what you need. You want to do whatever they tell you because you want the results they are selling! Then you've done it. You've done all they asked. But you're miserable, and you're exhausted. Either you lost the weight because you were so damn perfect, or you burned out before you made it to their "finish line." Either way, when the dust settled and you were left to yourself again, eventually, everything returned to "normal" and you were right back where you started. All the old habits came back, and the weight you lost came along with those old habits. In the fallout of your last fad diet, did it ever occur to you that maybe you hadn't failed the diet but the diet failed you? The truth is, you were not the problem. The diet was.

I know what it's like to think "I'm the problem," or "I'm just not enough." For me, it showed up most often when I went bra shopping. (Sorry, guys, a little girl-talk here for a moment; just skip this paragraph if you need to.) Ladies, bra shopping sucks! It especially sucks for someone like me who was never busty except when I nursed my babies. All my life, I've been pretty "slight of figure." There's a lot of shame and embarrassment that bubbles up inside me even talking about it, but I share this with you because for me, bra shopping is a lot like dieting. I go into the department store and NOTHING FITS. I can't fill out anything on the rack. My bust size is not even on the charts. It doesn't exist. So I ask you, have I failed? Am I just not woman enough? Hell, no! It took me quite awhile to make peace with it, but just like dieting has failed you, department stores failed me! It wasn't until I discovered a T-shirt bra on Amazon that I finally found my happy place. I found what worked for me. I don't bother with department-store bra shopping anymore. I'm done with it! And now I know that I was never the problem; the department store was.

Dieting for health is a lie. It was never designed to give you lasting results. It was never intended to bring you joy in your journey. It's a modern torture chamber we have all been brainwashed to think is a necessary part of life. **To weed out the myths and lies of diet culture, it will take repetition. Go to the toolkit and download Diet Culture Truth Bombs to read through some reminders about the problem with diets. You can print these out to read regularly, or write them on your bathroom mirror, or make yourself flashcards or a bookmark.** These will help you start to focus more on health, and less on weight. Diet culture does not need to run the show anymore. The good news is that there is another way.

So read on. You are going to pick up the pieces and put something beautiful in its place. You are going to learn to trust yourself again and crowd out all the old diet-culture programming.

TOOLKIT:

- PDF—Diet Culture Truth Bombs

CHAPTER 2 JOURNAL PROMPTS

1. What is your history with dieting? How many have you been on? Which ones? What worked and what didn't?

2. How has diet culture changed the way you think about health?

3. How has dieting affected how you think about food?

4. How has dieting influenced your thoughts and feelings about yourself?

5. What do you most want to leave behind from diet culture? What would a better way of moving forward feel like for you?

3

The Life You Want

HAVE YOU EVER BEEN STOPPED IN your tracks by someone asking you why you want to do something? WHY can be one of the hardest questions to answer, but it is also the most important. At first blush, when you ask yourself why you want to become healthier, it may be all about losing weight. Maybe you want to feel more comfortable in your own skin. Maybe you crave more confidence when you walk into a room. In this chapter, we're going to dig a little deeper so we can ground you in your unique reasons for reclaiming your health. You're going to discover that there is more to this than a new dress size. Much, much more.

As long as your reasons for moving forward are weaker than your reasons for staying put, you will never begin. Do you remember the story of Bilbo Baggins from *The Hobbit*? He was well off in his cozy little cottage in the Shire. He had all the comforts and amenities a hobbit could want. But was he happy? When Gandolf appeared offering the sheltered hobbit a chance for adventure, Bilbo had to weigh how happy he really was with his comforts and conveniences. He had to consider how much joy and satisfaction a quest across the valleys and mountains would bring him. Ultimately, Bilbo left behind what he thought made him happy and chose to seek something more. There's a difference between happiness and joy. Happiness focuses on convenient gratification and comfort. Joy, on the other hand, goes deeper.

Joy comes from satisfaction in a job well done and lasting personal fulfillment.

So, I ask you, are you happy? Are you REALLY happy? Are you satisfied with where you are and where you're headed? As hard as it is to admit, I hardly think you would be reading this book if you believed you were already living your best life. Let's redefine what it means when you say you are happy. Let's start aiming higher. Let's shoot for joy.

There's a comedian my family and I love named Brian Reagan. He has a monologue where he goes to his doctor, and his doctor tells him he needs to lose some weight, etc., etc. As Brian is walking out, the doctor makes one more sweeping statement: "Oh, and Brian, no more dairy." Shocked and flabbergasted, Brian says the doctor might as well have said, "Oh, and Brian, no more happiness." While this comedy sketch always makes me and my family laugh out loud, there's a part of me that cringes at what it's really saying. Are we so attached to a particular indulgence that we think it is the root of our happiness?

As you explore your WHY with me in this chapter, please be willing to be honest with yourself about what would truly bring you joy. Once you are clear on what you really want out of life, you're ready to explore your WHY. What are you in this for, anyway? What is this health journey really about for you? In this chapter, we will not stay on the surface of happiness. We will dive into who you are, why you are here, and what you are meant to do. It's only when you know these things that you can truly feel that the journey ahead of you is worth the sacrifice of the status quo because you know it will bring you joy.

What If?

I take every new client through a process of exploring their WHY. If you want a similar experience, **I have created a guided visualization where you can craft your Wellness Vision. Getting crystal clear on your unique WHY—your unique vision and purpose for health and wellness—will set the tone for the rest of your journey. Take a moment to pause and go to danielledinkelman.com/tool-**

kit to download the workbook and watch the video to create your personalized Wellness Vision.

It's time to paint a picture of your future life. No, not with a paint-brush. Just in your mind and with your words. The more you really close your eyes and see it for yourself, the more powerful it will become, so be sure to go through this process in the *Wellness Vision* video.

What would your life look like if you were in fabulous health? What would you have that you don't have now? What would you be doing? How would it feel to be healthy and thriving? Health is a means to an end. What's your end purpose for wanting to be healthier?

Sit with these questions and journal on them as much as you can. Let your imagination explore this alternative universe where you are living your best life. Look for the things that really matter to you. For many of my clients, it's about being more active and enjoying time, travel, and adventure with their families. For others, it's about being well enough to better serve in their career, charitable pursuits, community, or church. Ultimately, it's about feeling joy.

You will find more joy and satisfaction when your life is aligned with what you deem most important. When the way you live aligns with your values, you will feel joy. I'm not talking about moral values or even "family" values. I'm talking about what really makes YOU light up. The things I value most in life and that bring me the most joy and fulfillment are authenticity, adventure, balance, intention, and personal development. When my life feels aligned with these values, I am living my best life. My Wellness Vision would paint a picture that has me living out these values. I know that when I am striving to live healthfully, I am more able to live this way. I bet the same is true for you. Take a moment to reflect on what you value most. Let those values guide the Wellness Vision you create for yourself.

So what about you? What does your painting look like? How does it feel to you? Feel free to go through the guided visualization as many times as you need until you are in love with the life you've envisioned. You know your Wellness Vision is right when it makes you say "Heck, yes!" Only then will you be willing to step out of your status quo to go make your vision a reality.

Putting Health On Autopilot

Many people never take that first step to create a healthy lifestyle because they think it's too hard. Once you have your vision firmly in place and compelling reasons for why you want to change, you are ready to explore how you will accomplish it. We will dive deep into this in chapters 5 and 6, where we talk about the work it takes and what makes that work doable. Here's a taste of what you can expect:

To illustrate, imagine you are a pilot. With your vision statement completed, you have locked in your destination: WHY you want to be healthier. You have every reason to press forward and create that healthier version of yourself. You know you deserve to feel vibrant and healthy because you have so much to offer. You are ready for takeoff.

So, what comes next? How will you make your vision a reality? You need lift. Once you get your plane in the air, your habits will allow you to put your health on autopilot. Initially, it will take some umph to get going, but you won't have to keep that up forever. If you follow the principles taught in this book, you will be able to intentionally design and execute a completely new way of living rooted in and supported by habit. More on this in chapter 6, but for now, rest assured that as you focus on habits, the work of getting healthy will become easier and easier.

Habits are your secret weapon. Once you understand how they work, how to change them, and how to create them, you will finally feel like the master of your own destiny. Your mission is not to become perfect. Your mission is to do the work to build the habits.

"But, Danielle," you might say, "it's impossible for me to change my habits. I've tried a hundred times!" I know it can feel daunting. Think of it in a new way, though. Imagine your habits are like riverbeds cut deeply into the earth. Your behavior is like water, following the course already made. In order to create a new habit, or riverbed, it will take some digging. You'll need to dig to reroute the water (your behavior) again and again until the new pathway is just as deep as the original. Repetition is your friend. Your behavior will become effortless and natural as you move in this new direction. What's more, you can build supports and dams to direct the water. In chapter 6, I'll show you what this translates to in real life. You will design a life that supports you in becoming who you want to become and live the way you want to live.

Now you get to trust me. Stick with me here. Keep reading. You'll see there is a doable, even fun, enjoyable way forward. Your vision is in sight. To get all the way there, you will need to learn to trust yourself again and embrace a new way of changing. I'll show you how.

Let's Talk about Trust

"I need to learn to trust myself again." I have heard this from many recovering yo-yo dieters who come to work with me on a new way of doing things. With chronic dieting comes chronic "failure," and that takes a toll on self-trust, big time.

In the science of behavior-change, there is a powerful concept worth considering at this point in your journey. You need to understand that how you feel right now about your ability to change is fluid. In behavior science, we call this "self-efficacy." Your confidence and belief in your ability to make changes and overcome obstacles is not fixed or unchangeable. Your self-efficacy CAN be strengthened. More on this in chapter 6, but here is the first thing you need to know: self-efficacy grows as you experience success. This is the key to your progress.

If success breeds success, we need to set ourselves up for it! We can rebuild our self-trust and confidence as we make changes in small and simple ways. It's okay to go for the small wins first! Keep your eye out for the low-hanging fruit. As you continue reading, pay attention to what behaviors your mind goes to when you think about your next steps. Find the ones that feel doable. "Shooting for the stars" is not the way to start if you want to set yourself up for success.

How else can you rebuild your trust in yourself? Well, when you choose a lifestyle approach rather than a dieting approach, you are no longer biohacking your way to a smaller pant size. Now you can make friends with your body. Your body is not your enemy; it is your ally. Slowly but surely, you can begin to trust the wisdom of your body again. In chapter 8, we'll be talking specifically about nutrition. You'll see that the more you focus on natural, wholesome foods, the more you can trust your body's hunger cues.

I know it's hard to imagine fully trusting yourself and your body again. Maybe you don't remember what it feels like to trust it. Perhaps the last time you didn't obsess over every little thing was when you were a child. Try to imagine or remember what that felt like. You can start with writing or repeating these affirmations: "I am setting myself up for success." "I am showing up for myself." "I am rebuilding trust with myself." "I am learning to trust my body."

It will come! With baby steps and small wins, you will feel your confidence and self-trust grow stronger and stronger. It has been said that "out of small and simple things, are great things brought to pass." Your health journey will be no exception.

Who Are "Healthy People," Anyway?

The idea of becoming healthier may feel like stepping into a new identity. Anytime we consider leveling up from our old self to our next self, we will face resistance. That is completely normal! In fact, if you start to feel a little panicked about changing your lifestyle, it means you're on the cusp of growth.

And please know that you don't have to trade your happiness for health. I am not a task master or personal trainer here to push you until you break. I will help you find that sweet spot between your comfort zone and panic zone. In between the two is your learning zone. To truly learn and grow, this is where you want to be as often as possible.

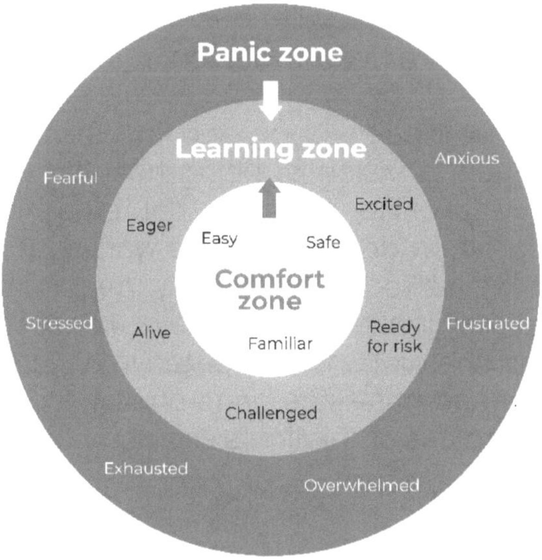

There's some muscle memory here. The brainwashing of diet culture may still be screaming in your ear: "No pain, no gain. "Go big or go home." "Big effort brings big rewards." You may still think you need to be in the panic zone. But here's the truth: Healthy living doesn't want suffering. Healthy living doesn't want dieting tactics. In fact, deprivation and dieting tactics DON'T WORK when it comes to healthy living.

Of course, there will be some hard work involved. It wouldn't be a transformation if it didn't take effort. But I promise we will be finding a doable way for you to make progress (more on that in chapter 5).

Healthy living is vibrant living. It requires showing up from a place of positive desire, self-love, intention, and joy. Anyone can choose to live that way now.

When I first started coaching, I worked with an amazing woman who is now a dear friend of mine. I noticed how, in our conversations, she kept using the words "healthy people" to describe what "those" types of people probably did. They were probably perfect. They probably had extreme discipline and on and on. Finally, I asked, "Who are these 'healthy people' you keep talking about?" We had a lengthy discussion about how she always put the runners, cyclists, and healthy eaters on a pedestal in her mind. It was also something she felt she could only achieve or become once her body changed so she could "look like a healthy person."

We challenged that idea head-on, and it was amazing to see what happened. My friend's vision of being healthy was strongly connected to being active. Her body was not releasing weight, and so she was holding off on doing what she wanted to do: compete in sprint triathlons. As we redefined "healthy people" by what they did rather than what they looked like, she said, "I choose to be a healthy person now." And she did! She competed in her first sprint triathlon shortly thereafter and has since gone on to fall completely in love with cycling, regardless of the limits she used to put on herself because of her body.

Now, I know not everyone dreams of being a triathlete. But I do think we tend to put the "result" we want on this unreachable pedestal. That's why I hope you have really enjoyed getting clear on WHY you want to be a "healthy person." I give you permission to start living the life you want today. Remember, finish lines are not a thing in the lifestyle approach. If you catch yourself thinking, "I'll be happy when . . ."—that's diet culture talking. No more putting off your happiness, your life's purpose, or next adventure until you reach some elusive result you have no control over. You can start living vibrantly *now*.

Habits Get Results

Whether it's a triathlon, international travel, or simply having the energy to keep up at home or at work, we all have results we hope to achieve. As you keep your Wellness Vision in mind, I want to tell you a little behavior-change secret: your vision is not your goal. As I alluded to before, the key to achieving your vision is creating habits that will lead you to it. We must focus on the habits and let the results take care of themselves.

In this book, you will learn how to set goals as part of your Wellness Blueprint. Setting goals in this way may be very different from how you've set goals before. Again, I want to emphasize that your vision is not your goal. In my lexicon, *goal* is synonymous with *plan*. You cannot plan to lose fifty pounds, but you can plan to create the habits that will lead to that weight loss. Do you see what I mean? There's a difference between setting an outcome goal and a behavior goal. I am much more interested in setting "behavior" goals because we can work on behavior. We cannot always control our outcomes.

Focusing too much on results and outcomes creates frustration. This is a journey, not a quick trip. Imagine if you hopped in the car for a twelve-hour ride and all you fixated on was your destination. How enjoyable would that trip be? You would probably be impatient with your fellow travelers, not rest or enjoy the scenery at all along the way, and not be happy until you got to where you were going. If that's how you road trip, I'd stay at home! Dieting is a trip to a destination. Lifestyle is a journey you enjoy.

There's some scientific modeling to support this way of moving through your journey toward your health goals. The Illness-Wellness Continuum developed by Dr. John Travis posits that "wellness is a process, never a static state."[4] Which is to say, there is no arrival. Also, it's not so much about where you are as it is about where you're headed. Which way are you facing? Are you headed toward illness? Or are you headed toward wellness? Again, it is about progress, not perfection. Even those who "achieve wellness" or those "healthy people" you may be putting up on a pedestal have to wake up every morning and make choices, just like everyone else.

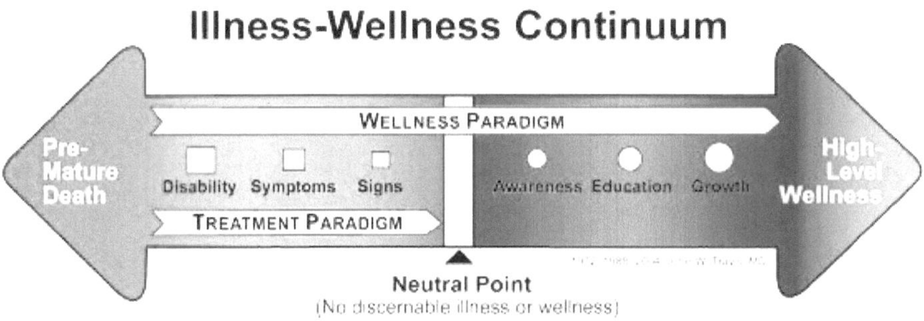

Remember that car accident I told you about? Well, even though I finally found some things I could do to be a functional human being again, I still deal with the effects of my neck and shoulder injuries on a regular basis. So do I consider myself a "healthy person"? Yes. Not because of what I have or the state I am in but because of the direction I choose to face every day. So, please, as you continue this journey, try to let go of results, finish lines, and pedestals. Instead, focus on choosing your daily thoughts, feelings, and actions. You can choose to show up and live as vibrantly as possible every day. One step at a time, you will move further and further away from illness and closer and closer to wellness. But what really matters is which way you face.

TOOLKIT:

- Video & PDF—Your Wellness Vision

CHAPTER 3 JOURNAL PROMPTS

1. List three things that would be different in your life if you were in perfect health.

2. What healthy habits would support you in becoming healthier?

3. What are the easy wins you could focus on to help you rebuild your trust and self-efficacy?

4. What do you most look forward to about being healthier? How can you start living that way now?

5. What result are you ready to loosen your grip on? What behaviors will you focus on instead of "over-efforting" your outcomes?

4

Yeah, But...

WHENEVER WE ARE AT THE THRESHOLD of something new, it is completely natural to feel resistance. It is normal to feel we have every excuse in the world to NOT move forward. In this chapter, we're going to get really honest with your "Yeah, buts." We will acknowledge them, sit down with them, and then invite them to leave, because you CAN do this, and you will.

Now, if I were personally coaching you, I would ask you how you feel about this new way of making healthy changes. Chances are, you may be feeling much of the resistance my clients have expressed. You may be feeling just as vulnerable and exposed as they do when they share their hesitations about moving forward. Let's address a few of those now.

First off, I know you've tried this before. "This" being a new beginning. Whether in the dieting or lifestyle arena, you've tried to make healthy changes many, many times. You might be saying to yourself, "What makes me think I can do this?" That's a great question. I invite you to sit with that for a bit. What emotions come up? What thoughts do you notice? (You can use the journal prompts at the end of this chapter to write them down.)

One of the biggest emotions you may notice is fear. I know this is scary to try again. Fear of failure is real. Fear of letting yourself down. Fear of letting others down. Fear of never, ever being successful and thereby never living the life you want. Those are some high stakes. Write down what is coming up for you, and just let yourself sit with those feelings for a moment. Don't worry, we'll let them go soon, but for now, let's look at them and be honest about them.

Now, as you write down the thoughts and emotions coming up about your new beginning, your body and your mind might be completely freaking out. Maybe your heart is racing, your body is jittery, and you literally just want to shut this book and walk away. That's okay. That's resistance. Keep breathing, keep reading, and let me help you through this.

When my fight-or-flight response alarm is going off in my brain and my body, I cup my hand and place my fingertips and thumb over my sternum in the middle of my chest and tap. Tapping this way and focusing on my breath will often calm my nervous system enough that I can think clearly again. Try it if you need some help getting through the rebellion your nervous system is mounting. **I made a video that coaches you through those thoughts and emotions. Go to danielledinkelman.com/toolkit to watch the video and get some help working through those feelings.**

As your friend and your coach, I have some thoughts for you to consider. First, I invite you to hold on tight to what made you want to try again. Remember your wake-up call. Remember the glimmer of hope you caught hold of. Remember your vision and why you want to see this through. Approach this with curiosity: "I wonder what will make the difference for me." "I am interested to see what will work for me this time."

One more thought for you. Maybe this time will be different because YOU are different. Maybe all the experiences, successes and failures you've had, have prepared you for this next step. You are not the same person you were ten years ago, one year ago, or even a month ago because you are continually learning and growing. Remember and realize you are not alone this time either. Before, you didn't have the guidance of this book. And if you feel you need more support and guidance than a book can offer, that's okay too. If you doubt your ability to do this alone—it means you're ready to ask for help. If so, please reach out! I can walk you through this process of learning and changing in one of my individual or group coaching programs. You don't have to do this alone. Getting a coach in your corner is a wonderful way to ensure your success. Tune in to what you need to be successful, and listen to that prompting.

But What If This Won't Work for Me?

Let's start reframing some of the thoughts coming up for you. Maybe there's just a whole lot of doubt. Does turning your health around sound like a fantasy? Okay, that's fine. For now, let's just focus on what's in front of you. Even if you try everything in this book and you don't lose fifty to one hundred pounds, you don't reverse your diabetes, and your anxiety never softens or goes away, is it still worth a try? The things you will learn in this book have no negative side effects. If it's not the weight, the diabetes, or the anxiety, I would put money on it that you will experience SOMETHING getting better as you focus on the healthy habits in this book. Consider that for a moment.

You may feel your situation is unique, and you may be wondering if this approach will really work for you. Of course your situation is unique! We can work with that. I hope you know by now that this book is not going to dictate your every move. It's not about "If you follow the Danielle Dinkelman Program to a T, your results are guaranteed." No! That's not what this is. Here, you will find powerful principles to heal yourself with lifestyle change. Every single application of these principles will be as unique as the fingerprint of the person applying them. So, please, make this fit YOUR life and YOUR circumstances. You are the expert on what will and will not work for you. You have complete veto power over any specific suggestions I offer in this book with one caveat—don't dismiss the principle behind the suggestion. Find a way to make it work for you.

Now, let's talk about failure. If you've failed before—GREAT! You've learned what does and does not work for you. That's the exact data we need to be successful next time. If you try and fail this time, look at it more as a learning experience. Take what you can from the experience, make adjustments, and move forward. If you need some hand-holding to walk you through that process, you know where to find me. Go to danielledinkelman.com to learn more about my individual and group coaching programs.

Consider this: all that resistance you're feeling as you step up to the plate to take your swing is setting you up for a great adventure. Have you ever watched a movie or read a book that didn't include adversity and opposition? Of course not! Those books don't sell, and those movies don't get made. Resistance is not a bad sign. It's a good sign! And you know what? YOU are the hero in your own story. You are about to embark on a life-changing, brag-worthy story. Every hero has a guide! Luke had Obi-Wan, Harry had Hagrid, and you've got me! Albeit a smaller, cuter, less-hairy guide—you've got a guide! I've got you, and you've got this.

Yeah But #1: Family

True or False? "My family wants me to be healthy and well." Of course, the people who love you want you to be healthier and happier, but at what cost, you might be thinking. So many of the women and men I coach worry that if they take the time and effort to make changes in their lifestyle, they are somehow putting their family out.

One of my recent clients felt that way. She was contemplating completely changing the type of foods she would feed herself and her family. She wanted to try more whole-food, plant-based eating. Her big resistance came in the form of a busy working husband and two young-adult and teenage sons. At least, in *her* head, this was her biggest obstacle. She worried about how they would feel about the change. She worried about the pushback they would give her. As she and I talked, we came up with some solutions. Sometimes the key to family resistance is simply having a conversation. She committed in our coaching session to talk with her husband and sons about the changes she wanted to make and WHY she wanted to make them. Of course, this went well because her family wanted her to be healthier and happier. They agreed dinners would now be different and if they didn't like what she made, they could hop in the car like the big boys they were and go get themselves a burger. A simple conversation focused on the real issues can put many concerns to rest.

You give so much to your family. When was the last time you asked for them to give something to you? It's okay to ask for and give yourself what you need to be happy, healthy, and whole. I wish every caring human would print in big bold letters on their bathroom mirror: "I can't draw water from an empty well." All the givers and doers in the world need to remember this! How can you give, give, give when you are depleted and drained? How can you keep giving when you are barely functioning? You can't. Filling your cup, and taking care of yourself is not selfish, it's essential.

Let's flip that on its head and examine it for a moment. Ask yourself: "How would my family benefit from me being healthier?" Grab a pen and paper and please write down at least twenty ways *you* taking care of *YOU* actually takes care of *them*. Think of the short term as well as the long term. You might be surprised at what you come up with.

When it really comes down to it, only you can take care of YOU. You take care of everyone else, so you are the most important person to take care of! Right? You may hear me say this a dozen more times, but it is possible that taking the time to care for yourself may be the most selfless thing you ever do.

Yeah But #2: Work

Next in line in the list of "Yeah, buts" is your job. You may feel you don't have the time or energy to focus on your health because of your busy career. "Getting healthier will be like a part-time job." Have you ever said this to yourself?

If you've never worried about that, you can skip this section. If you do worry that getting healthy will be too demanding, you might need to hang with me for a moment. Let's think about this. Could it be that what's good for your health is also good for your career? What do you think? Is that possible?

There is a lot of research on how the health and wellness of employees impacts productivity in the workplace. Simply google *presenteeism*, and you'll see impressive data on how much less productive people are, even though they are present at work, if their state of mental and physical health is lacking. Absenteeism and wellness is also well studied. We know that people who take good care of themselves get sick less often and therefore miss less work.

It makes sense, right? Of course our health and wellness impacts our productivity and being present at work. How you feel will affect every aspect of your life. You know that better than anyone. I know it too! Remember my auto-accident injury? I knew I could be a better mother to my two-year-old, but it was incredibly hard to do so with the pain I was in. We're only human. So let's take care of ourselves. I believe the people who depend on us at home and at work will be glad we do.

Sure, it may take some trade-offs to accomplish this, but what I'm saying is that it will be worth it for you and for your career. You may have to change one thing in order to get another. You may have to give up something you're used to so you can create a healthier new normal. I'll dive into more of these trade-offs in chapter 5, but for now, begin to believe that, whatever it takes, it will be time and energy well spent.

Imagine if you showed up to work at your best. How would life be better for you and for those you work with? What are some ways your customers or clients would benefit from you being in tip-top shape? Take some time to jot these down. It's powerful to connect the dots so you can give yourself permission to make your health a priority. Because let's face it, if you don't make your health a priority, who will?

Yeah But #3: Money

Here's another big "Yeah, but": getting healthy is expensive. What do you think? True or False? Are you holding back on beginning a concerted effort in becoming healthier because you're worried about money? That's understandable. There's a lot out there you could spend your money on in the name of health. There are gym memberships or home gym equipment, and nutrition systems and diet fees (but you already know we won't be doing so much of that here). Then there are meal delivery and buying healthy foods at the grocery store. And yes, you *could* invest in a personal trainer or health coach, but you don't have to be rich to remodel your health.

One way to look at it is to compare the cost of illness with the cost of wellness. Think of all the money you're spending on medications and doctor visits. How much of that would dissipate if you were in a better state of health? I've gotta tell you, when we changed the way we ate at home when my four kids were little, we went from seeing the doctor for coughs, sinus infections, and ear infections multiple times a year to hardly at all. Our immune systems get stronger as we take better care of ourselves! It is amazing.

Now, of course, money can make things easier when it comes to reclaiming your health. I'm a big believer in investing in myself because I know I am worth it. If I can find something or someone to help make changes faster, easier, or more effective, I will invest in that! I have invested in books, courses, and coaches for life, relationships, health, and business. I even have my own health-and-wellness coach because I believe in investing in myself. I am my greatest asset. I am worth the investment, and I always get a "return" on my investments in myself. That being said, you can build a healthy lifestyle on ANY budget.

One more thing to consider when it comes to health and money: How much is your current lifestyle costing you? How often do you eat out? Those restaurant bills can add up pretty quickly. How much money do you spend on treats and junk food? Those are some of the most expensive things on the shelves! How about soda? I have had clients who quit their multiple-times-a-day soda habit and found they had a lot of extra cash at the end of the week! They loved getting to use the money they saved on themselves in other fun ways. I encourage you to take some time to write down your current lifestyle and medical expenses. You'll see that adopting a healthier lifestyle won't cost you as much as it will save.

Yeah But #4: Self-Care is Selfish

Last thought. True or False: prioritizing my health is selfish. This one is so, so hard for many of my clients. Most of the women and men I work with are givers. They give and serve and give some more. Whether in their roles as a parent or grandparent or in their careers, it's hard for them to believe it is not selfish to take time and energy for themselves or spend money on themselves. Is this true for you? If so, you're not alone.

I get it. I used to have a hard time with this too. As a mother of four, I believed I was only a good mother if I spent every moment with my kids. I thought I was only being productive if I was taking care of them or our home. This was a pretty miserable way to live, and you know what? It wasn't really worth it. The more I took time for myself, the better caretaker and nurturer I became. The more I allowed others to support me and my family, the lighter my load was and the happier I felt. You know that phrase "If momma ain't happy, ain't nobody happy"? Well, it's so true. And the same goes for all women and men in a giver's role.

Whatever your "Yeah, buts," whether they be related to time, energy, or money, you can retrain your brain and move forward. Here are three things to start reprogramming your brain with: 1) Of course you are worth it! You are worth it because you are human. Every human on this planet, even the homeless and the destitute, have inherent value. Your value is not determined by your results or productivity in society. You are valuable because you are alive. 2) You deserve to be happy. I love that "the pursuit of happiness" is in the United States Declaration of Independence. Pursuing happiness is not selfish; it's an unalienable right! If everyone else has a right to pursue health and happiness, then why not you? 3) You deserve to take up time and space. You have needs. You have wants. It is okay to have your needs and desires met. Of course, anything can be taken to an extreme, but chances are, if you're self-conscious about taking time, energy, and money for yourself, you're not at risk for taking so much for yourself that you leave the people you care about with nothing.

If you're struggling with any of these mindset shifts around taking care of yourself, go ahead and read this chapter on a daily basis. Open yourself mentally and emotionally to begin thinking and feeling differently about taking care of yourself. If you need to, think of taking care of yourself as a selfless act because in taking care of yourself, you are actually taking care of all the people who depend on you.

Now, as you step into a self-care mentality, let's move on to chapter 5, where I'll give you more details on what it looks like to reclaim your health with lifestyle. You'll get clear on the trade-offs required in this journey, and you'll be glad to know that this new approach always gives back more than it takes. I'm excited to continue this journey with you.

TOOLKIT:

- Video—Tapping through Resistance

CHAPTER 4 JOURNAL PROMPTS

1. What fears or excuses are coming up for you as you consider pursuing a healthy lifestyle?

2. What past failures are causing you to doubt yourself? What did you learn from those experiences that can actually be helpful for you this time around?

3. Who are you feeling would "lose out" if you took more time and attention for yourself? How would they actually be better served by you taking care of yourself?

4. What are the pros and cons of focusing on your health when it comes to your job and finances?

5. What mantra or "I am" statement will help you remember that you are worth taking better care of? Write it down and put it somewhere you will see it daily.

5

The Trade-Offs

RECLAIMING YOUR HEALTH WITH A LIFESTYLE approach will certainly take work. It will take sacrifice. I like to think of the effort and sacrifice as a "trade-off."

"You can't get something for nothing" is true in life and in health. If you want a different output, you need to change the input. That's the trade-off! Of course this is hard at first. We like to do what is familiar. Change is uncomfortable but not impossible, and it most certainly does not have to be miserable.

The reality of trade-offs is something I teach my children. My six-year-old was in the habit of staying awake late into the night to play. Consequently, he was also in the habit of being very cranky and sluggish the next morning, so I sat him down and laid out the trade-offs. "When you stay up too late, you feel tired in the morning. If you don't want to feel tired in the morning, you need to go to sleep when it's bedtime." It took three or four days before he really started listening to me. He wanted to make a different trade-off. He wanted to stay home from school when he was too tired! Of course, that wasn't an acceptable solution.

We do this as adults, don't we? I know I do! We want to have our cake and eat it too. But the truth is, we have to face the natural consequences of our choices. When you pick up a stick, you get both ends whether you like it or not. If we want a different output, we need to make a different input. So the first step to better health is getting clear on the choices and consequences—our habits and the results. Only then can we choose differently.

We can't *not* change our habits if we really want to get healthy. That might be hard to swallow, but that is one of the trade-offs. That's the reality of human behavior and health. The good news is that you have help. Chapter 6 will give you all the behavior-change strategies you need to be successful.

Sometimes it's hard to be honest about where our past habits and lifestyle have brought us. But you can be honest about what needs to change without shaming yourself. I like to remind my clients (and myself) that they did the best they could at the time. You can love, forgive, and accept yourself and move forward. The up-side of all this is that if our past choices created the problem, our future choices can create the solution.

What Will It Take to Reclaim Your Health?

The principles of a healthy lifestyle are the same for everyone. It's the *application* of these principles that looks different for each individual. The trade-offs you need to make may be different than someone else's. In this book, we'll focus on five crucial areas of healthy living:

- Sleep
- Nutrition
- Exercise
- Stress Management
- Mindset

Each area will be laid out in greater detail in chapters 7 through 11. For now, let's take a bird's-eye view of them. As you think about these five areas of focus, ask yourself: What do I need to stop doing? Then ask: What do I need to start doing? What trade-offs will you need to make in each area? Remember, the goal is to feel better, more vibrant, and healthy so you can show up as your highest-functioning self. Listen to your intuition here.

A word of caution: if you are already feeling overwhelmed, that's okay. You might be looking at the five areas and say, "I need help with ALL of them!" That's fine. We can work with that. Remember that everyone hikes Mount Everest the same way: one step at a time. That feeling of overwhelm is a sign of taking on too much all at once. Pace yourself. Don't look at the summit and beat yourself up for not being there yet. You're here for the adventure and the journey, remember? You'll get there when you get there. So think of it like putting one foot in front of the other. What comes first? What's directly in front of you now?

A helpful container to put around this first step of your journey is to think only about the next ninety days. What is reasonable for you to focus on in the next ninety days? Start there. You don't have to have all the answers right now. In this book there's a chapter for each aspect of your healthy lifestyle to guide you through the process. And remember, you don't have to jump into action right now! Just keep reading. Soak it all in, and all the tools and strategies I am giving you in this book will be here when you're ready to move into action.

Speaking of which, now is a good time to introduce a pretty important perspective as you consider changing your habits and lifestyle. The Stages of Change[5] is a behavior-change model developed by James Prochaska and Carlo DiClemente. The following graphic reassures us that changing behavior has more than two stages: changing and not changing. There are actually five stages. You can be at different stages in different areas of your life. You could be in the Action Stage for prioritizing sleep but the Precontemplation Stage for improving nutrition. That's okay! The other important thing to note is that the stages can be quite fluid. You can move back and forth between stages, and you can also get bumped down all the way from stage 4 back to stage 1. Life happens! This model of change gives us perspective on that process and reminds us that we can learn from each relapse. That's the key: you're making progress as long as you are learning.

I share this because I hope you will be patient with yourself. You are a complex human being living a complex human life. As long as you are supported and intentional, anything is possible; it may just take some time.

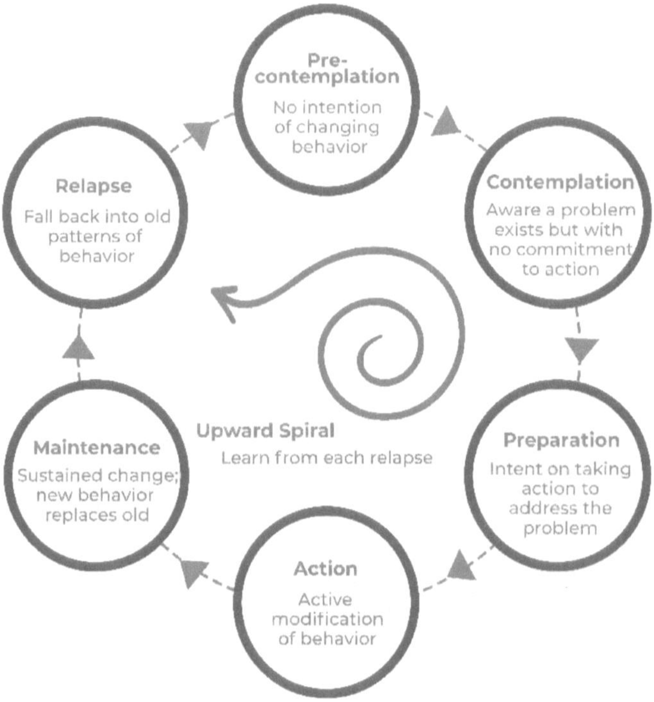

With that in mind, **let's consider what your areas of focus would like to begin with. Go to danielledinkelman.com/toolkit to fill out your very own Wellness Wheel and Health Behavior Baseline Quiz to get a clear picture of your starting point.**

Check Your Expectations

Now that you're getting some clarity on which areas of health and wellness you would like to focus on first, it's time to put all those "yeah, buts" we talked about in the last chapter to rest (or at least put them on the shelf). The reasons and excuses for not moving forward in your health goals will never completely go away, but I can give you some new language to use when these old buggers show up now and again. These are the trade-offs—letting go of the old to make room for the new. You'll be changing the input, so you can have a different output.

Most of the women and men I work with suffer from unrealistically high expectations of themselves. Whether it's in their work, family responsibilities, or personal life, they beat themselves up whenever they fall short. And let's face it, they almost always fall short because their best is never good enough (thanks a lot, Perfectionism). Their expectations are simply too high. If you can relate, this is a very good place to start.

If you expect to be perfect, you will be disappointed. Where do you expect perfection of yourself? Let's be real here. Pull out your journal to get clear and present with this right now. If you are willing to believe you don't have to be everything to everyone, you're in a better position to make the trade-offs necessary to take care of yourself.

Look at your life. Where are you giving more than you need to? Think of how you spend your time, energy, and money. Where is there room for adjustment IF you adjust your expectations for yourself? You know, in the business world, especially technology products, there's a concept in the industry called MVP—minimum viable product. Companies pushing the outer limits of technological advancement don't go out and try to create the PERFECT product, they try to create the NEXT product. MVP is not a bad idea when it comes to life's commitments of time, energy, and money. Where are you overdelivering? Where could you pull back just a bit?

Here's a tough one for a lot of my clients: Are you ready to start saying no without feeling guilty? To take back your time, energy, and money, you will need to say no to some people and things. Are you ready to stop feeling guilty?

You can be more realistic about your bandwidth. You are not superhuman—and that's okay! Because you have a finite amount of time, energy, and money, it's okay to make adjustments and trade-offs. Let's take a closer look at those trade-offs now.

Taking the Time

One of the biggest trade-offs you'll need to face is carving out time. Do you feel like there's just never enough time to do everything you need to do? Are you constantly rushing from one activity to the next? Do you feel like your schedule rules your life? It may be time to turn things around. If you feel victim to a lack of time, you need to put yourself back in the driver's seat.

For starters, refer back to your expectations. Remember that you do NOT have to do it all. Remember that you are done being everything to everyone. With that in mind, look at how you are spending your time and question EVERYTHING.

Have you ever tried the Marie Kondo method of purging your possessions? This famous closet cleaner and hoarder healer recommends not just looking at what you have and pulling out the things you think you can part with. No, she tells you to pull every single item out of the closet, the garage, the kitchen cupboards, or whatever area you are working on, and clear out the clutter. There's something pretty powerful about this process. What if we did this with our schedules? What if we pulled everything out, held it in our hands, and asked, "Does this spark joy?"[6] or "Is this essential to my purpose in life?" Big questions, I know, but this is where you get to start from scratch and redesign your life from the ground up. It's time to start living life more proactively, and less reactively.

How you spend your time reveals what you value most. Make a list or a mind map of all the responsibilities and activities on your plate. To make a mind map, write "me" in the middle of a piece of paper and draw a circle around it. Now, start drawing lines out to anything that you spend your time and energy on. Keep going until you've created a web with all your responsibilities and activities. Which ones reflect what is really important to you? What's missing? What do you wish there was more space for? What needs to go? Identify those nonessentials and cut the cord now before you change your mind. Write the email, make the phone call, let people know you are simplifying your life, and don't be afraid to let people down. They'll get over it.

There's a big difference between *finding* the time and *making* the time. It takes intention. It requires that you are crystal clear on your priorities. It requires you to make choices and trade-offs. This is what it takes to put yourself back in the driver's seat of your life.

One of the things that comes up most often around time management with my clients is taking time for themselves. Again, here is where the big-hearted, service-oriented women and men I love so much have a hard time looking at self-care as anything but selfish. Keep reframing this thought if it is still coming up for you. If you're ready to believe differently, it's time to put yourself on your to-do list.

I had a client once imagine her life was a pie chart. I asked her how much of each piece of the pie went to the various responsibilities in her life. She said 50 percent went to work, 25 percent went to her kids, and 25 percent went to her husband. It was a pretty eye-opening experience for her to put numbers and percentages to it like that. As a coach, it's just my job to ask the right questions, so, of course, I said, "Where is the time for you?" Her answer was obviously, zero percent. From there our work was clear. We needed to make time in her life for HER. We worked on adjusting the expectations she had for herself, as well as the expectations she believed her clients and family had for her, then went to work carving out 5 percent here and 5 percent there until she felt she could say about 20 percent of her day went to taking care of herself. It was wonderful to walk her through this process. You can do the same!

What parts of your day will you set aside just for you? What will you do with that time? What do YOU need? You might be used to thinking only about what others need, but if you are truly going to take a lifestyle approach to reclaiming your health, you get to start tending to *your* needs as well.

Investing in Your Health

Another big trade-off you might need to make is using your money to invest in your health. If your relationship with money is not healthy, it will be hard to invest in yourself.

Have you ever thought about your relationship with money? Maybe that's a funny way to think about it, but money is really no different than time. It's a finite resource you get to choose how to use. You decide whether you will be a victim to it or the wise steward of it. Sure, this is easy for people who have plenty, but even if you feel you have less than the ideal amount, how you think and feel about money will actually make a huge difference in your reality. If you focus on how there's never enough money, you'll be right. If you focus on how lucky you are to always have enough to meet your needs, you'll also be right.

While most of my clients don't struggle with what has been coined as "money mindset," I definitely have fought that fight myself. I like to think I am winning. I am making progress, and I am in a better place with my relationship with money than I have ever been. If you feel you could improve how you think and feel about money, keep reading. If you don't struggle with this, feel free to skip to the next section of this chapter.

When it comes to your relationship with money, there are three things to be mindful of: facts, feelings, and choices. Let's look at facts as they relate to money and your health and wellness. Facts will include:

- Your income
- The number of people in your household
- The cost of your home, car, groceries, etc.

When we look at facts, we can definitely find things to shuffle around. Budgets can always be reimagined. Just like your time or your closet, chances are there are things you can clear out to make room for what is most important to you.

One of the biggest hang-ups I see people have around money and health is the cost of food. They believe healthy food is expensive. So here's a fact for you: if you do it right, truly healthy eating actually SAVES you money. As you'll see in chapter 8, the more natural, wholesome foods you eat, the lower your grocery bill will be. I'll show you in more detail when we get there.

Let's look at your feelings around money. Do you feel it is okay to invest in yourself? That's a hard one for a lot of people. Money, just like time, is for taking care of everyone else, not me, they say. There's that fear of selfishness coming up again. Think of it this way: what would your ROI, or return on investment, be if you invested in yourself? One of the biggest returns is the possibility of getting off expensive medications or preventing the conditions that would require them. Strengthening your immune system and going to the doctor less as we discussed in the last chapter. What else? Maybe the return is not financial. Maybe it's emotional, maybe it's better relationships, or maybe it's physical. Maybe feeling better in your body is ROI enough. Are those things worth it to you? We spend money on things like this all the time! Why not on your health and well-being? Something to sit with and consider.

Now, let's talk about choices. Money, like time, is something we get to choose how we spend! Step back and really see yourself as the decision-maker in your life when it comes to money. Again, it's time to put yourself in the driver's seat. There's no right or wrong way to manage your money. There's no right or wrong way to invest money in your health and wellness. What is important to one person may be completely nonessential to you and your situation. Maybe it is absolutely essential for you to acquire an at-home treadmill. Maybe for another, there's no need because they live near a park and the weather is always seventy degrees! We are all in unique circumstances, so we get to make unique choices.

Where can you improve your relationship with money? How can the facts, your feelings, and your choices help you make space for what you need to do to reclaim your health? I'm proud of you for considering what needs to shift for you.

This Is Worth It

I hope you are beginning to feel that it is okay to take the time, energy, and money to take care of yourself. This is where success starts for every one of my clients: when they really capture this new belief that it's worth the trade-offs; when they want it and know they deserve it; and when they believe it doesn't have to be as hard or impossible as they thought it was.

By small and simple things you CAN change your life and your health. Refining and rearranging how you spend your time, money, and energy will make all the difference. With this, you are doing the work and making the space to take care of yourself. It will be worth it! These small decisions will make a big impact over time. You'll be setting a wonderful example for your friends and family. You'll soon be feeling more vibrant and healthy, and everyone who depends on you will notice the difference. Everyone wins when you do what it takes to take care of yourself.

At times, the trade-offs may seem like too much to ask. That's okay. It's normal to feel like that. I invite you to just experiment with trade-offs if you need to at first. I had a client tell me she was tired and exhausted all the time and didn't know what to do. She was a mother of six with two of her little ones home with her all day. When I asked if she ever took a nap in the middle of the day, she scoffed. However, we couldn't think of anything else to help her have more energy, so we got creative. She made a plan to take a nap when her little ones napped, even though she would be giving up her chance to clean the house. I'll never forget what she shared with me in our next coaching session. She tried it, and it worked! The nap helped her feel much better during the latter part of her day, and she was able to show up as the mom she wanted to be for her older kids. She admitted her house was less tidy, but she said, "For how good I felt, though, I'll take that trade-off!" What will you give to feel that way? What will your trade-offs be? It will take time for you to recognize them, and it will take some creativity to find new ways of doing things, but I assure you, it will be worth it.

More trade-offs will become apparent to you as we go along. I can't wait to walk you through those five crucial aspects of healthy living. In chapters 7 through 11, we'll dig into sleep, nutrition, exercise, stress management, and mindset. Keep an eye out for what YOUR trade-offs in each area may be. Remember, the name of the game is doable and enjoyable. Please do not continue reading this book, bracing yourself to do whatever I tell you to do. Just learn the principles of reclaiming your health and follow your intuition on how exactly to go about applying them in your life. Before we go there, though, there's one more thing you need to be successful. You need to know HOW to make healthy changes in sustainable ways. This is where the magic really happens.

TOOLKIT:

- PDF - Wellness Wheel
- PDF - Health Behavior Baseline Quiz

CHAPTER 5 JOURNAL PROMPTS

1. What parts of your day will you set aside just for you? What will you do with that time? What do YOU need?

2. List all the "priorities" and responsibilities you have in your life. How balanced does your life feel between these priorities and responsibilities? What could you do to take some pressure off?

3. Create a mind map of all the activities you spend time on. Which ones are in line with your top priorities? Which ones could you let go of if you needed to?

4. Take a look at your income and expenses. Make a list of expenses that would vanish (or decrease) if you adopted a healthier lifestyle? Tally up the total potential savings.

5. What work will be required of you to create a healthier lifestyle? What sacrifices will you need to make? What benefits do you expect to receive in return?

6

This Makes It Doable

MOST PEOPLE DON'T LIKE CHANGE. OTHER people crave it! It is the difference between people who are born and raised in the same town and never leave and those who can't stand to stay in the same place for more than a couple of years. How does the word *change* make you feel, really?

Whether you believe change is fun or hard, chances are, changing your behavior is much different than moving to a new city. Most of us know very little about how to actually transform our eating habits and health. I blame diet culture. Whether we've been a yo-yo dieter for years or have just watched our friends and family get on and off that roller coaster, the only model for change we have is the all-or-nothing approach of fad dieting. There's a huge problem with this. Dieting tactics don't work for lifestyle change. By nature, they are only intended to get you through the next six weeks (or however long the diet is supposed to last)!

In this chapter, you will learn how to let go of that misguided approach to behavior change. No more white-knuckling healthy changes. There is a better way. There is a more doable, enjoyable way. In this chapter you will learn:

- How to navigate the ups and downs

- What a habit actually is
- How to change old habits and create new ones
- How to not burn out along the way
- How to support the new habits you make
- How to know you're on the right track

Where did I get all this? Well, let me give you a little backstory here. I'm one of those people who when I decide I'm going to change something, I just do! No more processed food? Done. Going to start running? Let's do it! Yoga? All right. I naturally knew how to make sustainable changes. The more I talked with others about it, though, the more I realized that this was not easy for most people. When I became interested in helping others to be successful in healthy lifestyle changes, I felt stuck. I knew how I made changes, but how could I help others do the same? I knew and respected the difference in personality types and personal histories and how that affected our ability and preferences for making changes. I knew what worked for me, but how would I know what would work for others? That's when I got my answer. Call it a "tap on the shoulder," divine intervention, or whatever you like, but I believe I was led to exactly where I needed to go and what I needed to learn to get the skills and expertise to help others make changes.

I was guided to one of the best health-and-wellness-coaching schools in the country. I completed the primary and master levels of certification, then went on to study for the national board exam for health and wellness coaching. For a year and a half, I studied the principles of behavior change and practiced powerful coaching skills like motivational interviewing and appreciative inquiry. Finally, I had a clear framework and science to understand and validate the way I had been making changes all along. The more I learned, the more I was convinced I had struck gold. If everyone else could come to understand the behavior-change science and had the right support and guidance along the way, we could ALL be successful in turning our health around with lifestyle!

I've been testing this theory for the last three years, and I am convinced everyone is capable of sustainable change. It has been amazing to see client after client reframe their approach to change, and with the support and guidance along the way, be able to progress in their journey.

My ultimate goal for you is the same goal I have for each of my clients: to help you do the work to build habits that will last. Only then is the effort worth it. Only then are you creating *sustainable* change. Habits are the key. In this chapter, I want to help you fill your toolbox with what you need to understand behavior change. Changing habits takes effort. Tools make it doable. The tools I'll give you here are the same tools my clients practice with every day. Once they really learn and apply these principles of behavior change, their journey becomes so much easier. I know they will help you too!

Sustainable Change

For a healthy lifestyle to work, it has to be *sustainable*. If I had a nickel for every time I used that word, I would have a lot of nickels. So what do I mean by sustainable? No, I'm not talking about sustainability in the environmentalist sense. I mean sustainable as in "capable of being sustained." So we're talking about behavior that's continual, viable, feasible, unceasing, livable, and supportable. Why is sustainability so important? Because lifestyle medicine only works its magic over *time*. Sleeping more, eating well, exercising enough, managing stress, and having a positive mindset can work miracles in your life—but only if you stick with it for a good long while.

So, what makes healthy change sustainable? In order to live healthfully for the long haul, you must find a way to *enjoy* the journey. Let's face it, humans don't keep doing what they don't enjoy. We're wired to seek pleasure, avoid pain, and conserve energy. These facts are things we need to work with, not ignore.

Set your sights on a sustainable lifestyle change. Sustainable equals enjoyable, and enjoyable equals sustainable. Commit now to make this work for you in a way you would enjoy for the rest of your life. No more suffering, deprivation, or misery.

Now, this does not mean you are committing to be perfect. By choosing the lifestyle approach to reclaiming your health, you most certainly will experience lapses and setbacks. As you try to change old habits around sleep, nutrition, exercise, stress management, and mindset, you will slip up. You will go back to old habits. Hear me now—that is totally okay. Remember the Stages of Change from the last chapter? Do you remember the part about setbacks? We "learn from each relapse." Failure is just a bump in the road if you keep moving forward. So that's all you have to do: commit to learning from each setback and continue moving forward. Perfection is not required.

When you mess up and slide back into old habits, you may be tempted to think, "Oh, great, now I am back to square one." The truth is that you're not! There's no such thing as "square one." I'll tell you why. Because each time you come back to try again, you are wiser. You know what worked and what didn't. In fact, every time you "fail," in some ways, you're more likely to be successful the next time you try. As cliché as this may sound, the key is to learn from your mistakes. It will take patience and commitment to do this. With a little bit of guidance and a whole lot of grace, you CAN change your life and health. Let's dive in.

Leveraging Habits

The primary tool at your disposal in your quest for sustainable change is the power of habit. Habits may be your enemy right now, but you can make them your ally. There have been volumes written on what habits are, why they run our lives, and how we can change them. Deepening your understanding of habits is vital to your success. You'll learn all the essentials here in this chapter.

Why is it so hard to DO what we KNOW we should do? Why is it so hard to kick a habit? One of the first things you must understand about habits is that habits operate from the subconscious part of our brain, the basal ganglia. This part of the brain is dominated by instinct. Habits are like computer programs that are encoded into our brains, often without us even realizing it. In fact, with every habit, there is more to it than just the thing you're doing (the behavior). There is also a trigger, something that initiates the habitual "programming," followed by the behavior itself, resulting in some sort of payoff we crave. This is explained beautifully in *The Power of Habit* by Charles Duhigg. Once we understand there is more to a habit than just the behavior, we can use these three parts to diagnose and redesign existing habits or use them to build completely new ones.[7]

Did you know that about 43 percent of your daily behavior is habitual?[8] That's nearly half of everything you do, day in and day out. Eating, sleeping, talking, working, parenting, driving, cleaning, and everything in between is largely driven by habits, not conscious decisions. Think about the last time you tied your shoes. Which laces did you tie first, your right foot or your left? Chances are you'd have to actually start tying your shoes to find out because it's not a conscious decision you make every day. It's a habit!

Why do habits run most of the show? What is the biological purpose of having so much of our lives run subconsciously? Well, think about it—our big brain has plenty to worry about already. Can you imagine if you had to take conscious thought for all the functions of your body? What if your heart only pumped and you only breathed in and out when you consciously thought about it? None of us would have lived this long, right? The idea is the same for the rest of our usual behaviors. Our brain is essentially always looking for ways to put daily tasks on autopilot. Remember, our brain is wired for survival. On this planet, survival means: seek pleasure, avoid pain, and conserve energy.

A few things happen when you recognize just how much of your behavior is driven by habit: 1) you stop blaming yourself so much, 2) you look at it as a puzzle that requires trial and error to solve, 3) you can focus your energy on creating habits in such a way healthy living becomes part of your subconscious programming.

So, repeat after me: "Habits are my friends!" Habits hold the key to creating a sustainable lifestyle by putting healthy behaviors on autopilot. To take charge of your habits, you'll need to practice being more aware of the triggers, behaviors, and payoffs inherent in your daily routines. Then you can put strategies in place to interrupt old habits or create new ones. **I have created a Habit Change Journal printable for you to coach you through assessing and changing your habits. Access this and all other bonus resources at danielledinkelman.com/toolkit.** With the Habit Journal, you'll be able to take stock of your habits and routines, design experiments for change, and reflect on your progress.

What do your habits look like? What are your triggers? What are you craving that keeps each habit alive? Keep your eyes open, and you'll start to recognize more and more just how powerful habits are in your life. You can't change what you can't see. Start with becoming more aware of the habits that are running the show.

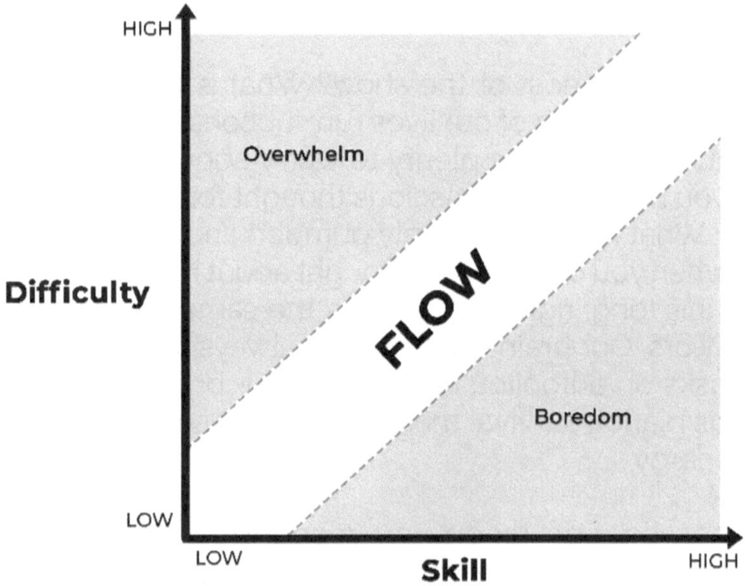

Finding Your Flow

I know changing habits can seem like a lot of work. You're not wrong! So how can we do what it takes to change our habits without burning out? The best burnout-protection tool I have to share with you is the flow finder. Most people think "getting into flow" is just for working on a project, but it can also be beautifully and effectively applied to habit change. Flow theory states that there is a balance point between the skill and the difficulty of an endeavor. When you continually stay "in the zone," you move onward and upward as your skill and the difficulty increases.[9] To do this, you must avoid boredom on the one side and panic or overwhelm on the other. By balancing your skill with the challenge you're taking on, you can avoid falling into either one. Put simply, if you want to stay engaged in your goals without being overwhelmed by them, find your flow.

I can always tell when a client is struggling to find their flow. Goal setting stresses them out! If you hate setting goals, it's a sign that you're doing it wrong. Diet culture strikes again if we are still thinking we need to set huge "go big or go home" sort of goals. No. Every time I go through a Blueprint Session with a new client, I know we've set the perfect focus areas and ninety-day goals for them if the goals feel both exciting AND doable. Doable + Excited = Flow.

As you move through the process of creating your Wellness Blueprint and then putting your plan into action, you may feel your balance point or your flow state come and go. As things get harder and obstacles arise, you may feel like you are being stretched to your limit. I call this your "edge." I recently met with a client who had tried the lifestyle approach on her own and failed. She told me she knew why it didn't work last time. It got too overwhelming. So we talked about respecting her edge this time around. I told her, "This time, lean into your edge but go no further. There's a sheer drop-off on the other side." We want to know where our edge is but not push past it. The last thing you want is to try so hard that you burn out.

The key is to set doable goals. When you think of goal setting, you may think of the popular SMART-goals framework. You know: specific, measurable, achievable, relevant, and time-bound. I find that most of my clients, and almost all recovering yo-yo dieters, have the hardest time with "achievable." They are so conditioned to force themselves into anything they are asked to do they have lost touch with their own opinion on what is realistic for them in the long-run. If that's you, you're not alone. It's okay to start with what feels doable. This is incredibly powerful for clients who feel like failures. Small wins with doable goals is what builds confidence. In behavior science, we call that confidence "self-efficacy." Albert Bandura coined the term, which simply refers to the level of belief we have in our ability to face a challenge or complete a task. Your self-efficacy may be dangerously low right now because of past failures. That's okay! Work with that and set a goal you know you can successfully accomplish. Start small and simple. Look for the low-hanging fruit. If your self-efficacy is moderate or high, set goals that feel doable and exciting for where you are at. Either way, it's good to keep a pulse on your self-efficacy so you can set goals accordingly. Continue forward in this way, constantly using your own built-in flow-finder: being mindful of your edge and intentional and realistic in your goal setting. Stay in your flow, and you will succeed.

Supporting Your New Habits

So, you've committed yourself to sustainable change. You understand how habits work. You're mindful of your self-efficacy and focused on finding your flow. You are light-years ahead of those trying to get healthy with lifestyle on their own. But there's one more tool you need to truly be successful.

The fact of the matter is that healthy habits aren't created in a vacuum. We have to find a way to be "in the world but not of the world." As much as we would like to, we can't escape our day-to-day life to go to a healthy-living monastery in the Himalayas and become health-nut monks. Trying to live this way can make you ultra-focused on willpower alone. Well, there's more to it than just depending on your willpower. You have to support the changes you make. More than depending on your own grit, you need to enlist support from the people around you, and you need to design your environment to support you as well.

When you ignore social support and creating a supportive environment, you may be setting yourself up for failure. That's working harder, not smarter. I know it's tempting to believe you need to just be strong enough to resist temptation and stay on the straight and narrow. Again, diet culture is to blame here. You may notice it's reflexive for you to blame yourself when you have a setback, but there may be more to it than that! Each time you have a relapse to old habits, you need to look at it like an experiment. Think objectively. When things don't work out, we can ask ourselves questions to check in if we are working smarter, not harder. Try asking questions like this:

- Personally: Am I having fun? Do I have everything I need to be successful?

- Socially: How can I enlist more support? Who is holding me back? How could they encourage and allow me to be successful more easily?

- Environmentally: Are my surroundings making it easier or harder to be successful? What could I redesign in my environment that would reduce friction and make healthy changes easier?

Ideally, you want all three areas of support working in your favor as much as humanly possible.

These are the sort of conversations I have with my clients on a regular basis. When we can answer these questions, we can see the gaps that need to be filled. When we get clear and intentional about leveraging all three areas in our favor, we can stop falling for the "just work harder" reflex. Maybe it wasn't willpower that failed when you weren't able to meet your goal of getting to bed at ten o'clock each night this week. Maybe there's a social motivation to stay up late because your husband or wife loves to binge Netflix on weeknights! Don't stop there. Notice what's influencing you and then do something to make things easier on yourself. Have a conversation! Enlist the support of friends and family. What could you ask them to do differently that would make this healthy change easier for you? Don't be afraid to ask.

What about environmental support? Your home, your car, your fridge, your bedroom, your neighborhood, all of these physical things make up your environment. Are they motivating you? Are they allowing you to follow through? Notice the friction in your environment and make adjustments where you can. Get the junk food out of the house. Tidy up before you go to bed so you wake up to a clean space and have no excuses to get out the door to go to the gym. Ignoring your environment sets you up for failure. Adjusting your environment to motivate you and allow you to make healthier choices helps you succeed.

Do you see where you set yourself up for failure in the past? What can you do to set yourself up for success? You can start working smarter, not harder. From now on, anytime you slip up, you won't throw in the towel, you'll just go back to the drawing board. Every perceived failure has something to teach you if you're willing to listen.

Permission to Choose Your Own Adventure

Now that you have the tools you need to make sustainable changes based in habits, you are ready to put it all into practice. This is where you get to step into the new belief that there is no one size fits all. You get to chart your course with the things you've learned in this chapter and the things you'll explore in the next.

Your starting point is unique to you. Reflecting on your Wellness Wheel from chapter 5, start where you *are*, not where you "should" be. The word *should* has no place in your health journey. This is your story. You get to choose your adventure and write your narrative.

Whatever your level of self-efficacy is, it's okay to take this at whatever pace you need to feel confident. It's okay to take this one step at a time. Work with what you've got, and that will be perfect for you.

As you take steps to change habits, be mindful of your edge. You'll know it when you see it. No more pushing yourself into anxiety and panic. Stay in your flow and keep moving forward.

A few more thoughts for you: don't leave your values behind (see chapter 3), and don't smother your personality in the name of progress. Focusing on what matters most to you and leaning into how you naturally like to move through life will serve you well. Trust yourself to know what brings you joy and find ways to include that in your journey. If you don't already know your personality type, I highly suggest taking some time to get clarity there. I've worked with clients of all different temperaments, and it is always more effective to coach them according to what makes them tick rather than use a blanket approach. My lighthearted, social-butterfly clients are going to approach goals differently than my analytically minded clients. Right? Of course! The first will need it to be fun; the other will need it to feel purposeful. **If you want more clarity on how you move through life, I've put together a few of my favorite personality inventories on this PDF inside the toolkit. If you haven't yet, you can still access this and other bonus resources at danielledinkelman.com/toolkit.** This journey is yours. Let's make it feel that way.

If at any time along the way you feel like you're forcing it—it's time to check in. Remember my client who was trying healthy habits for the second time? When she feels like she's pushing herself too far, she tells me, "I'm on the edge." It happens regularly. I tell her it's great that she is recognizing that feeling. We talk through what she needs to get back into flow. For her, slight adjustments have made all the difference. If she starts feeling stressed because she doesn't have enough variety in the healthy foods she's eating, she makes a plan to find new recipes. If she is not feeling supported by a family member and their behavior is hijacking her best efforts, she commits to have a conversation with them to enlist more of their help. It's these small adjustments and consistent self-awareness that are helping her take steady strides forward. No more yo-yo. No more roller coaster. No more all-or-nothing. Just steady, mindful progress. This is what I hope for you as well.

As you continue reading, you'll see that the next 5 chapters are dedicated to each of the Five Keys to Healthy Living. Each chapter will help you tap into the what, how, and why of improving sleep, nutrition, exercise, stress management, and mindset. As you read these, know that you get to choose your own adventure. Refer to your wellness wheel when you feel ready to dig into setting goals, making plans, and experimenting with strategies for the areas most relevant to you.

TOOLKIT:

- Habit Change Journal
- Personality Profile Inventories

CHAPTER 6 JOURNAL PROMPTS

1. Look at the two or three areas of focus you chose from the last chapter. What stage of change are you in for each? What can you do to help yourself move to the next stage?

2. What unhealthy habits are running in your life right now? What healthy habits would you like to see in the future? (Download your Habit Change Journal" to create traction on changing/creating habits.)

3. When it comes to change, what feels doable right now? What will you feel ready for after that? And after that?

4. Choose one of your areas of focus. What conversations do you need to have to enlist support? What will you change in your physical surroundings to be supportive? (Download the "Six Source Change Plan Worksheet" to make sure you cover all the bases for each goal and set yourself up for success.)

5. How will your health journey be unique to you? Your values? Your personality? Your starting point? Your pace?

7

You've Already Got a Bed

MOST OF MY CLIENTS COME TO me thinking that if they can perfect their nutrition and overcome harmful eating habits, their health and wellness dreams will come true. The problem is that most of the people I work with have been through the wringer with dieting, and their relationship with food and with themselves is quite strained. That's why I start with sleep. It's a great place to practice putting yourself first, remodeling your habits, and laying a foundation for wellness. It is totally normal to feel overwhelmed, especially if you know you have low self-efficacy starting out. So when healthy living seems hard, start with sleep.

If you are focused on weight loss, you definitely need to consider how well you are sleeping. I have had clients who are eating absolutely perfectly and still not losing weight. Sleep can be the thing that holds you back from weight loss. Sleep deprivation has been shown to decrease that amount of weight a person is able to lose. If you want to set your body up for success in weight loss, do not skip this chapter!

How do you know you could do better in this area? The Health Behavior Baseline Quiz from chapter 5 will give you some insight.

It will show you what behaviors are strong or lacking when it comes to prioritizing sleep. You can also take a look at how you're feeling day-to-day. Here are some signs of sleep deprivation to look out for:

1. Moodiness, crankiness, irritability

2. Cognitive function lags (focus, forming thoughts into words, reasoning)

3. Insatiable appetite during the day

4. Fatigue during the day

How many of the above signs of sleep deprivation do you notice in your day-to-day life? Most clients notice these troublesome signs. They know they need to set goals around sleep in our coaching work. They see they are not showing up at their best. Sleep deprivation affects how they feel at work as well as how they are with their family.

One young mother I worked with a few years ago was so busy taking care of everyone else and having no me-time during the day that she sacrificed sleep to get her me-time in the evening. On top of that, it was hard for her to improve sleep because her kids depended on her for comfort in the middle of the night. With a willingness to implement new policies and routines for herself and her children, she was eventually able to get more sleep at night. She was able to find a place in her day for "me-time" and thereby have the energy to show up as her best self.

One businessman I worked with came to me looking for answers for how to sleep better. He could only get three hours of sleep a night. His body just would not sleep any more than that. After months of concerted effort perfecting his sleep hygiene and focusing on stress management, nutrition, and exercise, his body began to submit to more and more sleep at night. Finally being able to sleep more was transformational for his happiness and health.

Whether your lack of sleep is affecting your job or family, trust me, your friends, your kids, and your coworkers want you to be well rested. It will be well worth the effort and the trade-offs to give your body the sleep it needs. It's time to stop putting sleep on the back burner. Whatever your frustrations with sleep are, know they can be improved with focused experimentation and consistent effort. Are you ready to explore how to improve your sleep? This chapter will help you do it.

Why Sleep Is Fabulous (And Terribly Underrated)

What happens while you sleep? If you could look through a window at your body's activity during the night, you would be amazed at what you see. We know that sleep is the body's rebuild-and-recover time. Much of the work your body does to detoxify, repair muscle tissue, recoup from stress, and fight infection happens while you sleep.

If sleep is so fabulous, why do so many of us trade it for a little more work on our boss's project, a couple more episodes of that show on Netflix, or folding that big mountain of laundry? Is that the trade-off we really want?

When you are tempted to sacrifice sleep for something else, consider this - YOU—your body and mind—are your most valuable possession you have. You MUST take care of yourself, and prioritizing sleep is one of the most powerful ways you can begin doing that. It's time to stop wearing late nights and next-day grogginess as badges of honor.

Most of us who work late into the night think we're making great use of our time and being extra productive. But let's be honest. It's not worth it. Have you ever hit that wall where you feel your brain just shut down but you keep working through it anyway? How productive are you being, really?

What do you feel like the next day? Or a couple of days after that late night? Have you ever noticed the consequences of sacrificing sleep? If you feel constant fatigue, that is not okay. That is your body screaming at you to give it the rest it needs. If your mind is fuzzy and you can't quite form ideas into words, that's another cry for help from your sleep-deprived brain. Stop excusing brain fog as normal—it's not. The CDC estimates that one in three Americans don't get enough sleep.[10] So while you're in good company, that does not make it okay.

If you want to start putting your health first, consider sleep as the highest form of self-care. Sufficient rest is one of the best gifts you can give your body. It works so hard for you all day long. Give your body the rest it deserves so it can keep supporting you. What would life be like if you had more energy? Picture yourself clearheaded, full of energy, and ready to meet the day. Let's look at what will help get you there.

Sleep More. Sleep Better.

What do you need to do to get the sleep you need? With sleep, quality matters just as much as quantity. We need to look at not only sleeping more but also sleeping better. With the clients I've coached on improving sleep, it's usually one or the other. The quality of sleep can be assessed by how rested you feel the next day. Consider if you were restless through the night or if you slept like a rock for several hours straight. Quantity is obvious. How many hours of sleep are you getting? What time do you fall asleep, and when do you wake up? Altogether, what are your quality and quantity sleep? It's important to know which one you need to improve because the strategies will differ.

To improve your quality of sleep, you can work on improving your environment, clearing your mind, and creating repetitive routines to train your body to wind down and rest. Sleep hygiene—it's not what you think. A quick Google search will give you the CDC's recommendations for improving sleep quality.[11] Here are the basic dos and don'ts:

- DO have a consistent bedtime
- DO have a bedroom that is quiet, dark, and kept at a comfortable temperature

- DON'T keep electronics or TVs in your bedroom
- DON'T consume large meals, caffeine, or alcohol before bedtime
- DO exercise during the day to help your body fall asleep at night

If any of these jump out at you as needing improvement, there's your starting point. I have seen these simple recommendations make HUGE differences in my clients' sleep. Do not underestimate the power of sleep hygiene. Also, as I've watched many, many clients put these tips into action, how quickly they noticed improvement varied. I encourage you to be consistent and patient. Every human being needs to do these five things. Do not take them lightly. They will do amazing things for you in the long run.

A word to the wise: snoring is no laughing matter. It may be cute and silly on your kids' cartoons, but in real life, it seriously messes with you. If you are snoring at night, it could be a sign you have sleep apnea, which most definitely affects your quality of sleep. Again, please take this seriously and see a doctor. If you need to sleep with a CPAP machine, get one. Typically, sleep apnea is weight-related, and as your body becomes healthier, the snoring may subside. In the meantime, do what it takes to give your body the gift of a good night's sleep.

What about improving the quantity of sleep you're getting? This is where we have to start being honest about the rest of our lives. Our bedtime is usually a result of the many dominos that fall earlier in our day. Be willing to step back and look at the big picture. Your goal should be to get about eight hours. The CDC recommends seven to nine for most adults.[12] So what will it take for you to fit that into your schedule? Too many of us have slipped into excusing away our sleep. Six hours does not count as a good night's rest. It's time to nurture yourself in this arena. Your body will thank you.

There are the basics. If you know your sleep issues are more a matter of the mind, we'll get to that next.

"Healthy People" Do This

Healthy people make time for sleep. They make it a priority. But what if you carve out the time, show up for your date with your pillow every night, and it just never goes well? If your mind is racing when you lie down to sleep, that's just another habit, and habits can be changed. The sleep hygiene we talked about a minute ago can help with this, but there are a few other things you can do. Notice what your mind is racing about. Is it your to-do list? Is it rehashing your day? Do you feel worried? Anxious? Identify the thoughts and feelings that keep you up at night so you can design an outlet. This is where a blank notebook can be your new best friend.

Writing down whatever is on your mind before you go to bed can be very helpful. Think of it as a "brain dump," where you get it all down on paper so you can clear your mind and rest. Once you have an outlet for those nagging thoughts and feelings, it's just a matter creating a new habit for your brain around bedtime. Do whatever it takes to feel calm and peaceful at night. This will look different for everyone. Design an evening routine that eases your brain and body into rest mode.

If you've tried all of that and your body is still refusing to sleep, it's time to get real about chemicals. What you do throughout the day will affect your ability to fall asleep at night. Consider these four chemicals: caffeine (from chocolate, coffee, tea, and soda), sugar (from processed foods and treats), alcohol, and medications. If you're taking any medications, talk with your doctor or pharmacist and educate yourself on whether those meds might be impacting your sleep. Work with your doctor to find a solution, if possible. As for caffeine and sugar, we have more control over these substances. Consider finding ways to cut back on how much you consume and then be mindful of what time of day you could stop consuming those things so they don't impact you at bedtime.

Remember my client from chapter 6? While she was laser-focused on improving her nutrition and avoiding burnout a second time, she stumbled upon a lovely side effect. As part of improving her nutrition, she was adjusting her consumption of soda and sweets. To her delight, she started sleeping better than ever before! I love the overlap and ripple effect different aspects of healthy living have on each other. This could be a small but mighty change for you too.

Finally, if you're doing everything you can to give your body a fighting chance to get a good night's rest and you still feel groggy during the day, I give you permission to take a nap. Yes, a nap. I know what you're thinking—naps are for babies and old people. No, they are for people who need them! Taking a nap is not lazy or selfish. It is well worth the sacrifice of time and productivity during your day. It doesn't have to be long. A catnap can do wonders. I recommend lying down for a nap no later than 1:00 p.m. or 2:00 p.m. Any later than that and you may not be tired enough to fall asleep that night. Experiment and see how it feels. You may not need this forever either. Give this gift to yourself until your body starts sleeping better at night.

Do you see how all this is a collection of habits? It's all about priorities, time management, evening routines, mental and emotional patterns, eating/drinking tendencies, and so on. Take a look at your situation through the lens of habit change you gained from reading chapter 6. With that in mind, check out the specific change strategies for improving sleep in the next section.

Your Very Own Sleep Study

Have you ever looked into doing a sleep study? It's where medical professionals have you sleep in a special room and hook you up to all sorts of wires and sensors. As you sleep for one, two, or three nights in this laboratory, professionals glean all kinds of information on how well you're sleeping. Then your doctor can use this to make recommendations for improving your sleep. The problem with official sleep studies is they are very expensive and it requires you to sleep outside of your natural habitat. Whether you do a sleep study to tell you what's wrong or you notice signs of sleep deprivation yourself, the solutions are often the same. Everyone who wants to improve sleep must face the habits we've already discussed in this chapter. The clients I've worked with who had trouble with sleep improved it by the time we finished working together. By simply learning about proper sleep conditions, examining where you can improve, and putting new behaviors and routines in place to give your body a chance, you basically have your very own sleep study!

So, what habits do you need to create so you can sleep better? This may take some brainstorming and experimenting. Stick with it, and you will find the answer. I had a client I worked with for six months. The entire time, she struggled with fatigue throughout the day. We covered all our bases, and I mean ALL of them. She was doing everything right but was still exhausted and drained every single day. In one coaching session, it came up that her husband snores. Bingo! She decided to try sleeping with earplugs to see if that did the trick. Eureka! It made all the difference. Soon she no longer needed to nap during the day. She was finally able to sleep soundly enough at night that she had the energy she needed to feel fabulous all day long. If you're not sure why you're not sleeping well, take a step back and think outside the box. You'll find your answer.

As you work to make necessary habit changes, remember to set yourself up for success. Don't try to do this alone. Remember supporting the changes you make? How can you leverage personal, social, and environmental factors in your favor? Routines will be mostly personal, but the people you live with may also play a role. What conversations do you need to have to help you get to bed on time? Environment is so huge when it comes to sleep too. Again, take those sleep-hygiene recommendations seriously. When I moved my phone out of my bedroom at night, my mind was so much more calm and clear when I climbed into bed. It is so nice to not have that phone be the last thing I look at before I close my eyes. What could help you? Be willing to mix things up a bit and create a new normal.

What if you try something new and it doesn't work right away? Remember that the key ingredient for changing or starting a habit is repetition, repetition, repetition. When we repeat a behavior, it sends a signal to our brain that "Hey, I could make life easier by putting this on autopilot. Let's send this one downstairs to the subconscious department." Do the reps to retrain your brain. Clients who are used to watching YouTube videos in bed or lying awake solving the world's problems in their mind have actually created a habit for their brain and body. It will take time, repetition, and consistency to retrain your brain to associate bed with sleep. Make your bedroom a sacred space. Don't work on your laptop, watch Netflix, or do productive work in bed. Let bed mean sleep. These little changes will make a big difference for your brain and body. Stick with it and be patient, and your body will get the message.

As you chip away at this, make sure you celebrate your progress. Notice any subtle shifts—they're a sign that it's working. Have someone you can brag to and get excited with when you notice you're not as tired during the day or that you got seven hours last night instead of five. The more you amplify your success, the more you'll be committed to staying the course.

It's All Connected

I hope you are feeling excited about sleep! I hope you are finding pieces of the puzzle that are fitting into place for you. I hope you're ready to change your narrative around sleep—it's not a waste of time; it's one of the best things you can do for yourself! Sleep deprivation is not a necessary evil for getting things done. It's not worth sacrificing your health.

There's a reason I began with sleep. Even if you ONLY focused on sleep—imagine how your health would improve. Lack of sleep puts our bodies into a stress state, and we know that stress is the root cause of so many physical, mental, and emotional problems. And so it follows that when we're sleeping better, so many other things become better too. It's a domino effect. Being well-rested helps your body feel safe and cared for so it can release excess weight and respond better to good nutrition and exercise. Sleep is a wonderful way to recover from stress. As we've seen, the ripple effect goes both ways. If your body is not willing to sleep, more exercise, less stress, and better nutrition will give your body what it needs to be able to rest. It's all connected! Picture it like a web. You cannot tug on one strand without moving all the others.

So let's get tugging! If sleep was lacking on your Health Behavior Baseline Quiz from chapter 5, I hope you've found an idea or two in this chapter to help you. **To get crystal clear on where you are with quality & quantity of sleep, go to the toolkit and download your Personal Sleep Assessment. This is where you can lay out in detail where you're at now and consider how you could**

improve in the next 90 days. Never underestimate the power of prioritizing sleep. This has been the missing piece for SO MANY of my clients. Magical things happen when you are getting enough sleep. Make sleep your new non-negotiable. It will pay you back a million times over.

TOOLKIT:

- Personal Sleep Assessment PDF

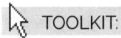

CHAPTER 7 JOURNAL PROMPTS

1. What benefits of better sleep are you most excited about?

2. Which area do you need to improve most: sleeping more or sleeping better? (Quantity or quality?)

3. What are three current habits that are holding you back from experiencing better sleep? What's one new habit that could help you improve?

4. What is your "low-hanging fruit" when it comes to sleeping better? What could you focus on doing or changing that feels most doable first?

5. How will sleep affect other aspects of your health and wellness? What other areas would you like to focus on that would make sleeping better easier? (Nutrition, stress management, exercise, etc.)

8

Eat Happy

HOW ABOUT A FRESH START WITH healthy eating? This can be a sticking point if you have a long history of yo-yo dieting, struggles with binge or emotional eating, food addictions, or eating disorders. I step into this topic with respect for all of those circumstances. I know nutrition can be a delicate subject. Seventy-five percent of the clients I have worked with over the last four years have come to me having been beaten and bruised by diet culture for years (some their entire lives). Let's be honest—most of us have some healing to do when it comes to our relationship with food and with ourselves. My intention with this chapter is to give you a fresh start with eating well. Let's wipe the slate clean and start anew. Forget almost everything you know about eating "healthy."

In this chapter, I share some very simple principles to guide your next steps with nutrition. You will find these points to be straightforward and, quite frankly, common sense. I'm inviting you to step away from all the hype, all the noise, and all the marketing out there. Quiet your mind and open your heart to see if the things I share with you ring true. Listen to your gut, your intuition, or whatever else you draw divine help and guidance from. These principles are true and good intuitively as well as intellectually. There is literally a mountain of research behind the ideas I will share with you. I encourage you to research them for yourself after I lay out the basics. Pure and simple. Listen, feel, and see for yourself.

Here's the first truth you need to know: food can create health. The right kind of food can even prevent and reverse our most terrifying diseases. I learned this shortly after losing three of my grandparents within three years. I watched them suffer as a result of dementia, stroke, heart attack, bypass surgery, and more. The entire time I witnessed their decline in health, I saw myself. I knew their genetics were my genetics, and it scared me to see how miserable they were as they deteriorated before my eyes. A year later, I had my eyes opened to the power of nutrition and the role it plays in our health outcomes.

After two years of studying every bit of information I could get my hands on about nourishing myself and my family, I learned there are ways of eating to prevent dementia, stroke, and heart attack. I learned you can reverse the harmful atherosclerosis that leads to myocardial infarctions (aka heart attacks) and the need for stents and bypass surgeries. This was mind-blowing to me because I had always believed genes determined my destiny, not my lifestyle. It was earth-shattering—and empowering. It was thrilling to know I could have a say in my health outcomes.

Before sharing the ins and outs of the power to heal your body with food, I want you to do something for me. Remember, the intent of this book is to make this journey doable AND enjoyable. So right now, let's start letting go of the limiting belief that healthy food is not fun, tasty, or enjoyable. Start believing healthy food CAN taste good! I am not here to strong-arm you into trading your happiness for your health. Quite the opposite. I'm inviting you to live in an abundant, joyful way AND reclaim your health in the process. Change will be necessary, but I believe it can be an enjoyable journey if you let it. Try to be open to believing you can have fun with this.

Finally, don't focus on how hard this is going to be. Let go of seeing reclaiming your health as an uphill battle. Your body is more forgiving than you think. It will thank you for every little thing you do in its best interest. Even if you have the worst of chronic diseases, even if you are morbidly obese, your body will thank you for nourishing it now. It will take time. It will take patience. But there will also be immediate responses you will notice from your body. Digestion, energy, joint pain, inflammation, sleep, and more will all begin to noticeably shift as you take care of this amazing body you are in. Even if you don't feel or see the impact of eating healthier right away, studies show there are immediate internal things that happen in response to the type of meals we consume. Trust in that. Trust that your body will know what to do with healthy food. One influential doctor, Dr. Michael Klapper, says, "You can be healthier with your very next meal."[13]

With a mind and heart open to a fresh start, let's look further into eating happily.

The Dose-Dependent Benefits of Eating a Little Better

From which type of ailments does your body need healing? Type 2 diabetes, high blood pressure, high cholesterol, atherosclerosis? What about arthritis? Sleep apnea? Autoimmune disease? Carpal tunnel? Joint pain? IBS, Crohn's, colitis? I have worked with clients with all of these and more. If not in relation to a diagnosed condition, maybe your desire for a healthier body is simple. You simply want to feel better. You want the energy you used to have. You want to feel light on your feet. You want to be able to move more freely and live more joyfully. Maybe that includes a little weight loss, or a lot. No matter what ails you, nutrition can help. Will it fix it? It's possible! While it's not a silver bullet, eating right definitely does a lot of the heavy lifting in health and healing. (But remember, nutrition is just one piece of the lifestyle approach to reclaiming your health.)

Your body will thank you for every step you take toward eating more natural foods. Many who advocate natural foods call it "whole-food, plant-based nutrition." I may use that term as well, but one big difference you will notice between me and others is that I don't care if you go all-in with this or not. I just want to encourage you to take ANY steps in this direction. Naturally, you will see the most dramatic impact the more you fully commit (I recommend working up to 90 percent of your nutrition being natural foods). But even if you go from 25 percent to 50 percent natural foods this year, your body will thank you!

Progress is progress. The longer you eat natural foods, the more your body will respond. (I'll share more on exactly what natural foods I'm talking about in a moment.) Anytime you use a lifestyle change to improve your health, you can trust the compound effect. The longer you do it, the greater benefit you will get. I suggest finding a way to enjoy eating as many natural foods as possible for the foreseeable future. I want you to design a new way of eating you can adopt for the rest of your life. (We're going to make sure you enjoy it!)

Some of the most important studies showing the benefits of natural foods were done in the field of heart disease. Two different doctors with slightly different approaches but working from the same idea found that heart disease could be halted, and even reversed, with nutrition. Dr. Esselstyn's and Dr. Ornish's work is foundational to the idea that the standard American diet leads to standard American diseases.[14] Heart disease is not an inevitability of aging, it's an inevitability of a lifetime of harmful nutrition. But when you look at the graphs in their studies, you see dose-dependent results. Even the patients who were partly compliant saw improvement. Of course, those who were most compliant experienced the most improvement. That's why 90 percent is the end goal. However, from a behavior-change standpoint, trying to do too much too fast may not be worth it.

Please do not take this exciting scientific discovery and dramatically change your diet overnight. To do so is to ignore the equal mountain of research in human behavior and habit change. It is far more important that you improve your nutrition while building sustainable, enjoyable habits around it. If you're up for doing this in a new way, and what I believe is a better way, you're in the right place.

You can absolutely turn your health around with food. There is no doubt about that. Let's just go about it in a way that won't freak you out. Do not use what you learn about whole-food, plant-based nutrition to deprive yourself to better health. No, no, no. You can nourish yourself to better health. No depriving, just nourishing. Diets can't heal, but food can.

Let's Not Overcomplicate This

What do I mean when I say "natural foods"? I choose that term because it's simple. The explanation can be simple, too, albeit very defined. As I've studied plant-based nutrition and the role diet has on disease, the ideal way for a human to eat boils down to two very simple parameters.

1. Eat mostly whole, unrefined foods. Avoid or minimize processed foods.

2. Eat mostly plants. Avoid or minimize animal products.

Whole foods are foods in their natural form or as close to it as is reasonable: whole grains, whole fruit, whole vegetables, whole legumes, and whole nuts and seeds. You can purchase or find these things in their whole, natural, edible form. You can cook them and eat them. You can blend them. All that matters is that you are consuming it in the way nature intended it to be consumed by humans. What about meat and dairy? Couldn't those arguably be considered whole foods? Yes! That's why the second question is so important.

The foods that heal are plants. You can think of it as five food groups: grains, beans, fruits, vegetables, nuts, and seeds. Picture it like this:

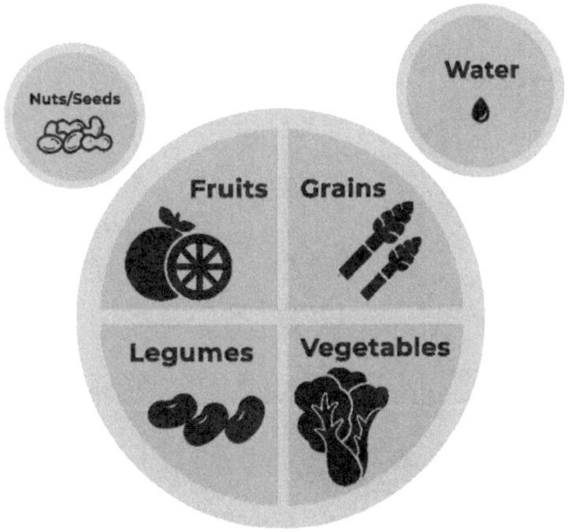

I know, I know, these are not your momma's food groups. I grew up with the food pyramid too! You know, where meat and dairy and oils were their own food groups! The more you research whole-food, plant-based nutrition, though, the more you will clearly see that plants are the way to go.

To have this explained in more detail, **go to your toolkit and watch the video Natural Foods Explained. There you'll see what it looks like to eat this way on a daily basis.**

I just want to get the clear and simple message across that if food is whole and comes from a plant, that's the food that will be most nourishing to your body. The foods that come from animals and processed/refined plants are damaging to your body. More on this in the video I mentioned.

One of the most important differences between plant-sourced and animal-sourced foods is that whole-plant foods have fiber. Animal-based foods do not. Fiber is only found in the plant kingdom. Did you know that only 6 percent of Americans get their daily recommended amount of fiber? That's pretty atrocious but not surprising. Our standard American diet is primarily refined plant foods (little to no fiber) and meat and dairy products (no fiber at all). It looks a little like this:

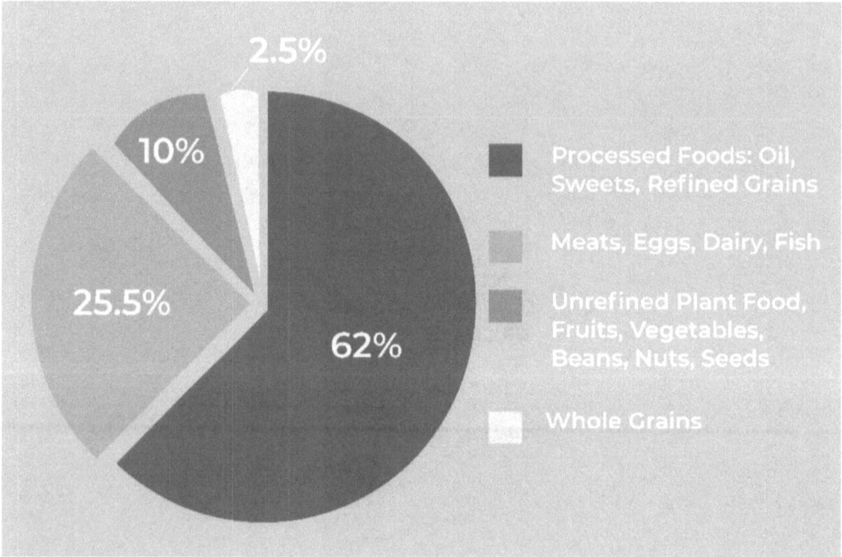

Pretty sad, right? Fiber is your friend. It keeps your body healthy. It keeps you regular! Fiber intake is associated with so many health benefits: decreased risk of heart disease, cancer, type 2 diabetes, stroke, and colon cancer.[15] We were designed to eat primarily plants. We were designed for fiber.

"But what about protein?" you might ask. Not to worry. Did you know plants have protein? Nuts, seeds, legumes, and whole grains have plenty of protein. Fruits and vegetables even contain protein! When we eat a balanced diet from all five *natural* food groups, we get the right amount of protein we need. **You don't have to stress about protein. Learn more about this in the video in your toolkit: *Why You Think You Need More Protein*.**

So what does eating this way actually look like? Don't worry, you don't only eat salad. There's more to it than fruits and vegetables. You will get full and have fun with the other food groups that complement the fruits and veggies. The whole grains, like rice, oats, quinoa, millet, amaranth, farro, and barley, are very satisfying and filling. They serve as the blank canvas for jazzing up your menu with flavorful herbs and spices. Beans are also very filling and full of fiber, vitamins, and minerals. Nuts and seeds can be soaked and blended and turned into creamy nut butters, sauces, creams, and dressings to be your new vehicle for flavor and fun. It's a new way of cooking and eating, and yes, it is fun, flavorful, and filling. **You can see the types of meals my family and I eat on a regular basis here in my five free recipes included in your toolkit, or take it a step further and purchase a copy of my four-week meal plan, available at daniellledinkelman.com/recipes**

Now that you're getting an idea of what to put on your plate, let's talk about how much. Remember my little truism: Eat whole foods—primarily plants, as much as you want.

What about portion control? The best news about eating natural foods is that you can eat when you're hungry, and stop when you feel full. When we eat natural foods, we can trust our natural hunger cues again. In fact, you might find you eat more food and more frequently when you choose to eat this way. Please do not apply any dieting tactics to this way of eating. Eat when you are hungry and stop when you are satisfied. Since these natural foods are high in fiber, and fiber is devoid of calories, you are eating more mass. Thus, you will get full without overeating calorie-wise. You'll practice listening to those hunger and fullness signals and find your new normal.

There is so much more to learn and explore in this universe of whole-food, plant-based eating. I encourage you to dip your toe in and see how it feels. **To keep you from being overwhelmed with the infinite resources you'll find, start with the ones listed in my Going Plant-Based Resource Guide (found in your toolkit) and simply watch the videos I mentioned.** That will be enough to get you started. As you experiment with eating this way, you will be amazed at how your body responds.

Food Choices Are Actually Food Habits

To truly leave diet culture behind and lean into a lifestyle approach to health and nutrition, we must remove shame. Responsibility is good. But not shame. Shame and guilt are in dieting territory, and you're not hanging out there anymore. I find it helps my clients to recognize it's not so much their food choices that have been running the show as much as their food habits.

There's no "just do it" here. We have to come at this with everything you know about how habits work (see chapter 6). So when you look at your life through the lens of habits, what habits are ruling the way you eat? Take a moment to get clear on that. We can work with wherever you are.

Many people I have talked to say, "Well, I'm a food addict." Forgive me, but I don't think calling ourselves food addicts is helpful because 1) it gives your power away, 2) it's a shaming label, 3) and it implies that something is WRONG with you and you are broken in some way. While the struggle is real, this is a disempowering way to think of yourself. Try this instead: "I am not a food addict. I've just been eating addictive foods." Here are a few more new thoughts to adopt:

- I can make healthy changes.
- I can get triggering foods out of my life.
- I can create new habits.
- I can be intentional about the way I eat.

Sometimes what you may think is food addiction is actually just emotional eating. This is extremely common in our culture because we deal with a lot of emotions and food is an easy access thing to use to deal with them. It goes a little something like this (notice the three parts of the habit):

1. You feel overwhelmed/stressed/angry/sad/lonely/ bored. (Trigger)

2. You go _____ and eat _____. (Behavior)

3. You feel calm/happy/fun/entertained. (Payoff)

That's all there is to it. Emotional eating is just a habit that intertwines feelings with food. You can unravel that when you are ready. You can simply replace the eating "routine" with a nonfood-related activity that gets you the same emotional relief.

Once you know what emotion you're dealing with and what you're actually craving (e.g., comfort, fun, etc.), you simply need to experiment with other things that satisfy that emotional craving. If you're feeling lonely, instead of reaching for the dark chocolate, call a friend. If you're feeling stressed and craving escape, go for a walk. If you are bored and craving fun, turn on your favorite sitcom. Find something that satisfies your emotional craving. That is how you conquer emotional eating—treat it like any other habit you want to change. Because that's all it is.

As you change your eating habits, remember that dieting tactics won't help with healthy eating. Review the old diet culture ways of thinking in chapter 2 and watch for when they start to creep into your mind. Now, let's talk strategy.

How Will You Feed Your Healthiest, Happiest Self?

Whenever you talk strategy for habit change, it's worth asking yourself where you want to end up. It's called "beginning with the end in mind." Where do you eventually want to be? Do you want to be eating 90 to 95 percent whole-food, plant-based? Or is your intention to just get to 60 to 70 percent? Either way, the approach is the same: you can rebuild your eating habits one layer at a time. Your end goal will keep you informed on how many more layers you need to go.

One of the most effective ways to slowly but surely adjust your eating habits is to work on one meal at a time. It's not helpful to snap your fingers and say, "Okay, today I start eating 100 percent plant-based!" Please don't do that. That would be setting yourself up for another roller coaster of go-big-or-go-home burnout. It's okay to start small and simple.

I find it's easiest for my clients to first focus on breakfast. Once they know how to prepare natural foods for that meal, they can go on to lunch, dinner, snacks, or dessert. The order is completely up to you! Whatever you do—do NOT white-knuckle this healthy-eating thing. We want to continually be working on what you are ready, willing, and able to change. Stretch yourself into your learning zone, not your panic zone.

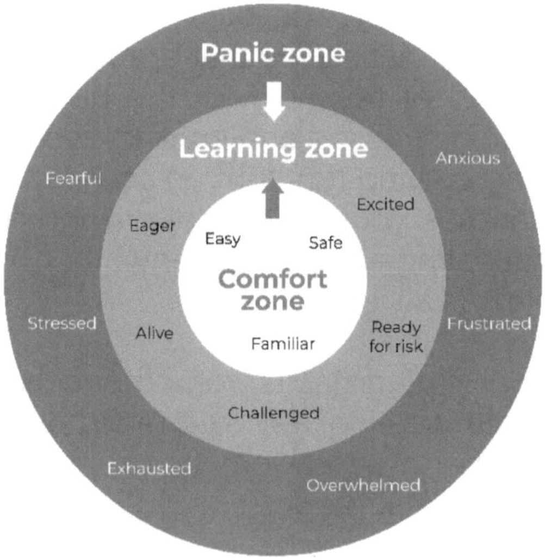

Find your "edge" and respect it. What do you *need* in order to stay out of panic? Does the food need to be easy to prepare? Does it need to be flavorful? Do you need a lot of variety? That's fine—you can do that! Do what you need to do stay in your "flow." Match your skill to the challenge. If it feels too challenging to start cooking and shopping a whole new way, do your homework and build the skills you need. You can also bring the challenge down a notch by lowering your expectations. Be patient in your progress. This is not a race. Walk—don't run.

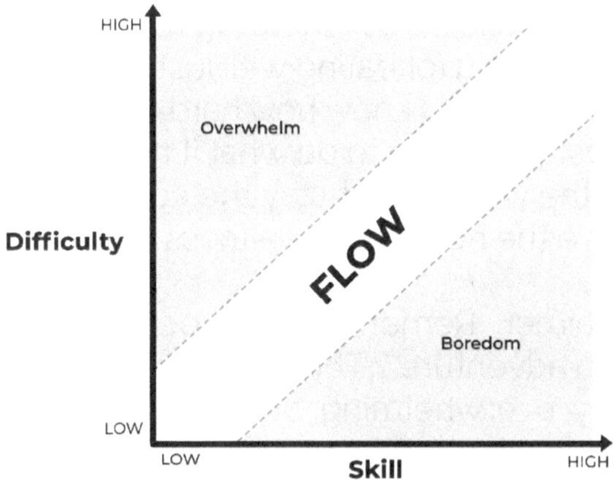

Once you decide what you will do, write it down. Make a plan and stick to it. Make sure it's doable and realistic. Make sure it's exciting and enjoyable. Draw your own line in the sand. Some of my clients start with "Okay, I'm done with cow's milk." Others start with going vegetarian and cutting back on eating meat. Whatever feels correct for you, go for it. And remember, with every step you take toward more natural foods, your body will thank you.

A Domino Effect You'll Love

Every aspect of health and wellness you work on, whether nutrition, sleep, exercise, stress management, or mindset, will impact the others. Eating well nourishes every cell in your body. As you slowly but surely improve the quality of your nutrition, you will notice changes in your body.

Celebrate every little change you feel. Notice how much better you are sleeping. Notice how much energy you have during the day. Notice how your mind feels clear and active. Notice how your relationship with food is getting better. You'll begin to see food as fuel.

Now, a word about weight loss. You may or may not experience weight loss right off the bat with moving to more wholesome, plant-based foods. Rest assured, this is totally okay. In my experience, about 50 percent of my clients experience weight loss immediately after changing their nutrition. Here is where we get to practice letting go of the myopic diet culture that ONLY cares about weight. Instead of stressing about weight loss, dig deep into your purpose, which is improving health. Please don't ignore all the other wonderful ways your body is thanking you for eating well just because the number on the scale isn't plummeting. I know how hard this can be, but I promise that if you can trust your body to do what it needs to, when it is ready to, it will release the weight. Just stay the course. The day will come when you will have the health and wellness you desire.

One more disclaimer: Remember the permission I gave you to "choose your own adventure"? This is where you get to do that. If nutrition feels heavy, overwhelming, and scary, it's okay to circle back to it later. I have had clients who were so wounded from their dieting history they did not want to touch nutrition with a ten-foot pole. That is just fine! You can choose another area of focus to start with. This will be true for you if your self-efficacy around eating healthy is very, very low. We can build that up with a sort of "backdoor" approach. Go to one of the other areas (sleep, exercise, stress management, or mindset) and start there. Build your momentum and confidence in those areas. You'll be pleasantly surprised at how that will help you feel ready to face nutrition later down the road.

Sooner or later, when you're ready, and at a pace you feel you can handle, you can make food your friend. Food is powerful. Food is medicine. Food is fantastic. When you're ready, you'll find that vibrant food builds a vibrant life. I'm excited for you to experience this. I'm excited for you to find your way to loving the food that loves you back. Wholesome nutrition is foundational to living the life you want.

TOOLKIT:

- Natural Foods Explained video
- Why You Think You Need More Protein video
- Going Plant-Based Resource Guide
- Five Plant-Based recipes

CHAPTER 8 JOURNAL PROMPTS

1. List three things you learned about healthy eating in this chapter. What interests you or excites you most about what you learned?

2. What percent of your current eating habits is whole-foods? What percent of your current eating habits is plant-based?

3. What healthy eating habits do you eventually want to adopt? How could you break those into individual steps you can work on over time?

4. What are you feeling ready, willing, and able to adjust in your eating habits?

5. What domino effect are you hoping for as you begin to eat better? (Better sleep, more energy, mental clarity, reduced pain and inflammation, etc.)

9

You Were Built to Move

HAVE YOU EVER REALLY STOPPED TO think about how wonderful your body is? Your body is AMAZING. It does so much without you even realizing it. Think back to high school biology. Can you name all the systems in your body? Just for fun, google "human body anatomy and trivia." Just a moment reviewing the facts leaves me in awe of the amazing gift this body is. It breathes, pumps blood, holds me up, and lets me do the things I need to, day in and day out.

If you've "been there, done that" with diet and exercise, you may have a hard time feeling grateful for your body. In the past, perhaps you have felt like your body is not your friend. Of course, nobody's body is perfect, so it can be easy to be hyper focused on all the things we perceive are wrong with our body.

Sometimes I struggle with this too. For me, it always comes back to that car-accident injury. Sometimes I feel like my body is still punishing me for that one big mistake. For my clients, it's the excess weight they can't ever seem to be free of, or the diabetes or high blood pressure or some other disease that ails them. Maybe you feel like your body has turned against you. When we step back from the negatives, though, there are always positives. You're still breathing, aren't you?

If you tend to think negatively about your body, I invite you to start practicing a little more gratitude for the gift it really is. You can even take a moment right now to place your hand on your heart, close your eyes, and talk to your body. Thank it for how it's supporting you. (I know, it's a little silly, but go with me here). When we can "love, forgive, and accept" ourselves and our body just as we are right now, we have the power to move forward.

Once you feel a little friendlier toward your body, maybe you can start feeling friendly toward the idea of exercise. Have you been in the doctor's office and he's looking at you over his thick-rimmed glasses and clipboard, asking how much exercise you're doing? How many times have you given the standard American answer? We laugh to ourselves and think—nope! Who has the time to exercise? The only people who exercise are those crazy marathon runners and bodybuilders, right?

It's for this sort of history that it's sometimes helpful to reframe our language. If the word *exercise* makes your lip curl with disgust and contempt, let's create a fresh start. Let's call it something else! Let's redefine exercise. You can call it "being active" or just "movement." Whatever it is you need to create a new start with moving your body more, let's do it.

Let's not only redefine exercise as something of your choosing, let's also reimagine what constitutes exercise/movement/activity. Exercise options are endless! Just because your doctor says you need to move more doesn't automatically mean you have to go get a gym membership. In this chapter, I want to help you explore how you can ENJOY being active and moving more. Like everything else in this book, it's absolutely essential you find YOUR way of doing this. Only then will you like it enough to make it part of your vibrant lifestyle.

There's More to Exercise Than Weight Loss

Have you known anyone obsessed with cars? I was raised by a car enthusiast. My dad was an auto mechanic, so as a kid, I was used to hearing him go on and on about the parts and features of different cars and trucks. The twinkle in his eye when he talked about the classic black 1972 Mustang he bought after high school is priceless.

My dad is one of those people who drool over the roar of a well-built engine. They itch to get behind the wheel and drive these machines just for fun. If you've ever driven a really well-made car, you know the feeling. You know the rush of laying down on the gas and feeling the power literally at your fingertips. It's exhilarating!

Our bodies are no different. If you were to give my dad back his high school dream car, do you think he would just let it sit in the driveway and say, "Oh, I just don't have time to take it out"? Did you know that it actually damages a vehicle to not drive it regularly? It's true! You'll kill the battery, stagnant oil and moisture buildup will corrode the engine, and the tires will lose air and flatten to the point they can no longer be used. Cars were not meant to sit in driveways, and bodies were not meant to sit all day either. Not moving your body enough is like owning a muscle car you never drive. It's just silly!

A sedentary or inactive lifestyle comes with risks and consequences. Just look at this from the World Health Organization: "Sedentary lifestyles increase all causes of mortality, double the risk of cardiovascular diseases, diabetes, and obesity, and increase the risks of colon cancer, high blood pressure, osteoporosis, lipid disorders, depression and anxiety."[16] The WHO is going so far as to name inactivity as one of the top ten causes of death. In fact, 60 to 85 percent of adults fit the bill when it comes to a sedentary lifestyle. Scary, right? Well, I know it's one thing to look at these global statistics, and it's another to look at your life and try to make changes. But that's okay. That's why you're reading this book, right? I've got you covered. Before we get into how to make this doable and enjoyable for you, let's dig a little deeper into the benefits of exercise.

When you move more, everything gets better! With exercise, you can prevent and manage disease, maintain a healthier weight, sleep better, have more energy, have a better mood, and even improve your sex life. So why not? In spite of how you feel about exercising, which of these benefits are most motivating to you? Write them down and keep them in mind as you make plans to become more active.

When I started exercising, it was for the mood boost. Shortly after I started going to my new massage therapist, I became pregnant with our second child, a little girl. I continued seeing my massage therapist throughout the pregnancy until at thirty-four weeks, the baby stopped moving. It was a Sunday morning in 2010. I sat through church waiting, watching, and panicking as I sat in the back pew scanning my watermelon-sized belly for any sign of life. I finally couldn't take it anymore and decided to go to the hospital. The nurses got me into a room and they put the all-too-familiar goo on my tummy and started using the handheld Doppler to search for my baby's heartbeat. There was nothing there. She was gone. Later that night I delivered a beautiful baby girl. She had long slender fingers and toes, a whole head of strawberry blonde hair, and skin as smooth as silk. But she never took a breath. She didn't open her eyes and look at me. I never got to hear her cry. This loss was beyond devastating. When I returned to my life and eventually to massage therapy, I was now not only broken on the outside but now on the inside too. I was overcome with grief that manifested as depression and anger. These emotions were heavy and insatiable, like a physical hunger pang that could never be satisfied. My massage therapist recommended running, not only for my auto-accident injury but for my emotions. I needed an outlet. And Lord knows I needed some endorphins! Running became my grief therapy. It gave me a place to think, a way to move my anger and my confusion and my sadness through my body. It probably saved my life.

Becoming active does not always have to be for physical reasons. You can have many reasons to start moving more. I've had clients who set exercise goals because they knew it would help with their depression or anxiety. Other clients set exercise goals because they know being outside in nature is a huge stress reliever for them. Whether it's a physical, mental, or emotional motivation, find a way to activate that desire to move your amazing body more. Use the gift God has given you. Enjoy it, have fun with it, nurture it, explore, and get out into the big wide world with it! You'll be very glad you did.

Let's Move More Because You Want To

So, can we agree it's a good idea to move more? Of course, but how will YOU start moving more? If regular exercise is not a part of your life, we first need to look at what sort of exercise you would like to do. Oh, and if you are exercising a little bit, I suggest looking for a way to up the ante. If you're walking every day, that's great, but let's get some more vigorous exercise in the mix too as soon as you are able. Before I dive into guidelines and recommendations for types of exercise, remember, the name of the game is ENJOYABLE exercise. Please don't do this because you know you "should." Do it because you want to. If you don't want to, find something that helps you feel more desire.

To truly enjoy exercise, you need to either enjoy and crave the activity itself, appreciate and yearn for the payback it gives you, or have a companion activity you look forward to. Netflix can be a great workout buddy. Podcasts, audiobooks, or your favorite music can be just the thing to get you out of bed and into your workout routine. Whatever you need to do to enjoy moving more, do it.

As you consider what type of exercise to choose, be sure to keep your unique values and personality in mind. If you're the social type and value meaningful connections with people, maybe you could work out with a friend or family member. If you value fun and variety, maybe a gym membership with all access to high-energy group classes would be your thing. If you're the fiery, driven type, look for something competitive or just intense enough to make you feel like you're doing something big and awesome. If you're analytical and logical, choose an activity that lets you track your progress and set new personal bests. These are just some ideas. You know yourself best. Get out there and find "your thing." Make it a priority to choose a workout that fits your personality so you're more likely to enjoy it.

Be mindful of your rebellion reflex as I share some recommendations for exercise. Remember that meme I mentioned? "I was going to do that, and then you told me to." Isn't that the way we humans are wired? We do not like to be told what to do! It needs to be our own idea. If you can find something you genuinely WANT to do rather than something you SHOULD do, you'll be much more likely to do that thing. That being said, here are some general guidelines to help inform your exercise goals.

Official recommendations from the U.S. Department of Health and Human Services state that "to attain the most health benefits from physical activity, adults need at least 150 to 300 minutes of moderate-intensity aerobic activity, like brisk walking or fast dancing, each week. Adults also need muscle-strengthening activity, like lifting weights or doing push-ups, at least 2 days each week."[17]

Translation? This can look different depending on how often you exercise. If you're going to exercise five days a week, shoot for thirty to sixty minutes a day. The guidelines specify, "Most activity can be aerobic, like walking, running, or anything that makes the heart beat faster." That's a great place to start. What can you do to get your heart rate up for thirty to sixty minutes?

Including resistance training is powerful, too, so don't overlook it. Body-weight exercises, including yoga and Pilates, could fit the bill here, or any kind of weight-lifting or resistance training.

If you don't know what to do to meet these guidelines, start small. Walking is a great way to start. But then do some brainstorming and do some research. What activity would really bring you joy and add some adventure and excitement to your life? We'll go there next.

Take On a New Identity

I believe Aristotle is credited with saying, "You are what you repeatedly do." One of the fun things about bringing more exercise and activity into your life is that you get to take on a new identity. You can become anything you want to be. Do you want to be a hiker? A bodybuilder? A cyclist? A runner? A roller skater? A rower? A rock climber? Sure, maybe you start with walking at first, but doesn't it sound fun to work up to really trying something new? Is there something you've always wanted to do but haven't?

For a few years, my husband and I talked about trying cross-country skiing. After all, we live in Utah and all the license plates here say, "The best snow on earth." Finally, after years of dreaming about it, we got a babysitter on a Saturday morning and went on our first ski date. I fell head-over-heels in love with cross-country skiing that day. (And yes, I did fall flat on my back a few times too!) It felt amazing to use my body to ski all over those trails. I loved being out in the pristine white snow surrounded by pine trees and a crystal blue sky. The best thing was the quiet. It was the most peaceful, exhilarating thing I had ever experienced. Now I'm hooked. I stay active all year so I can be in shape for ski season. I've become a skier.

I hope you're daydreaming about something you can work toward. I hope you're thinking of something you can genuinely enjoy, even just a little bit.

Once you decide how you'll be more active, be careful not to "should" all over yourself. It's okay to take a little time to put a new exercise habit in place. You don't have to start a routine overnight. You can be strategic about adding exercise to your life. Return to chapter 6 with exercise in mind and see what you need to do. You'll need to think about what you'll do, how often, how long, and at what time of day. Maybe you'll need to get some workout clothes or other equipment. Maybe you'll need to choose which gym you'll go to if that's the route you want to take. Do what you've got to do and pat yourself on the back along the way as you prepare to start moving more.

The name of the game is repetition. Routine is the key to becoming active and fit. The more you go and the more you enjoy going, the more it will become a part of your new normal. Put in the reps by showing up.

As you work through creating a new routine for yourself, please don't beat yourself up when you slip up. Just get right back to it the very next day. Stop blaming willpower and start building a habit. We'll talk more about supporting your new exercise routine next.

Just Start (Today)

Nike says "Just do it." I say "Just start." You can start today. Getting the ball rolling is often the hardest part. Commit yourself to get started. Even if it's brainstorming, planning, researching, or preparing. You can start by going on a walk every day at lunch. You can start where you are, then take another step.

How you start will depend on what stage of change you are in. What stage of change are you in for exercise?

- Precontemplation: It's not on my radar.
- Contemplation: I'm thinking about exercising more someday.

- Preparation: I'm planning on starting within the next thirty days.
- Action: I have been exercising regularly for less than six months.
- Maintenance: I have been doing it for more than six months.
- Termination: It's not even work for me anymore to exercise regularly. I just do it without thinking about it.

Wherever you are, the goal is to move yourself to the next stage. As long as you're progressing through the stages, that's all that matters. If you're in termination for exercise, you can hop to the next chapter.

Identifying the stage of change you are in is very helpful for pacing yourself. I often see this with my clients. People tend to decide what they want and then expect themselves to jump right into doing it. This usually ends badly because they are basically skipping the preparation stage and trying to go straight from contemplation to action. Pausing to assess where you are in the stages of change will give you clarity on where you are and what comes next. Use the stages of change to pace yourself. Give yourself permission to decide what you want, then identify the steps of getting there.

Once you're in action on your new exercise routine, be mindful of the feeling. Humans keep doing what they enjoy, and they stop when it's not worth it anymore. I don't want you to fall into that trap, so watch out for yourself. Remember flow theory? Use overwhelm and boredom as your two guideposts. If you start to feel either, make an adjustment! If you're bored, mix it up or add something to make it more fun! If you're overwhelmed, how can you make it feel more doable? Beware of overwhelm and boredom and stay in your flow. Like driving a car, you've got to keep your hands on the wheel so you can be making fine-tuned adjustments in your course. No over-correcting! Just stay on the road.

Now, a word about fitting exercise into your busy schedule. I have never met anyone who "finds" time to do anything. People who decide to make changes in their lives MAKE time for what they deem important enough. If this has been a struggle for you, you'll need to make room in your life for moving more. Remember the idea of trade-offs? You may need to clean out your schedule a bit so you have ample time to do what matters to you. Taking care of yourself and "getting the car out of the driveway" matters. If this is a sticking point, revisit chapter 5 and do some journaling on what you need to do to make time for an exercise routine.

Above all, let's do this on your terms. Don't do this like someone else would; do it like YOU would. There are a million ways to have an active lifestyle. You're going to need to think outside the box and follow your own path on this one. All that matters is that you are moving lots and loving it. **You can start by printing this one page list of 103 Ways to Move More from your toolkit. Skim the page and cross out any you know you would absolutely hate. Circle the ones you've done before and could enjoy getting back to someday. Highlight the ones you might be interested in trying out. From your circled and highlighted items, write down 3 to 5 that you want to explore in the next 90 days.**

Endorphins Make People Happy

With each aspect of your healthy lifestyle, I hope you always come back to WHY you're doing it. I can spend all day telling you about the great health benefits of exercise, but YOUR reason will be unique to you. So what is it? Why are you going to commit to moving more?

I'll tell you why I really exercise every day—it's the endorphins. Man, those endorphins are good stuff. Reese Witherspoon's character in *Legally Blonde* had it right: "Exercise gives you endorphins. Endorphins make you happy. Happy people don't shoot their husbands. They just don't!" But seriously, for me, my mental and emotional health DEPENDS on that daily dose of feel-good hormones. The physical benefits are secondary. That's my why.

My active lifestyle has taken on a lot of different forms over the years. There was a time when all I did was run and do yoga. Then I became interested in weight lifting. I read three books on the subject and went all in. About a year later, I explored cycling. Oh, and then jump rope! Talk about a fun way to get your heart rate up—once you get good enough you're not slapping your arms and legs every two seconds. Nowadays I am doing a hybrid of them all. I make sure I do thirty minutes of brisk walking or jogging or stationary bike or jump rope. Then I throw in some weight lifting once or twice a week.

I make sure to do at least fifteen minutes of yoga every morning. And during ski season, you can bet I'm on the trails every Saturday morning until the snow dries up in March. Then I switch to a weekly hike. This is what I need to feel happy and fit and balanced. I am so excited for you to create your own active lifestyle, whatever that may be.

If you need another reason to start moving more, here's some food for thought: Moving more can make all the difference. For several of my clients, exercise has been the missing piece. They may have been eating really well for months but did not notice any change in their bodies, especially when it came to releasing excess weight. It wasn't until we put an exercise routine in place that they broke through that barrier. If you find you're at a plateau in your weight loss, look at how you can move more. If you're already exercising, mix it up and throw in something different! It could be just the jump start your body is asking for.

Another great reason for moving more is that exercise can be great "me-time." Or "you time." You understand what I'm saying. Time to yourself! Time to just be with yourself and move your body. What a gift! In this way, exercise is a form of self-care and stress management. It's healthy to take time to do something just for you. Exercise is no exception. The more you exercise, the more you'll notice changes in your physical health, but you'll probably notice changes in your mental and emotional health too. I hope you'll find a way to make this a part of your vibrant lifestyle and love it!

TOOLKIT:

- PDF—103 Ways to Move More

CHAPTER 9 JOURNAL PROMPTS

1. What benefits (mental, physical, emotional, etc.) of exercise do you need most right now?

2. Make a list of twenty activities you enjoy that get your body moving and heart pumping. Think outside the box! And for now, ignore ALL obstacles; pretend anything is possible. (Use the 103 Ways to Move More activity in your toolkit for inspiration.)

3. Picture your future self living an active lifestyle. Who are you? "I am a (runner, skier, hiker, swimmer, cyclist, gardener, bodybuilder, etc.)."

4. What stage of change are you in for beginning an exercise routine? What will you do to move through that stage and on to the next?

5. Write down your top three reasons for becoming an active person. Post them where you can see them.

10

You're Not Superhuman (And That's Okay!)

ALL TOO OFTEN, I'LL HAVE A client come to me saying they need help with nutrition and with exercise, but after a few weeks of focusing on those things, they realize the actual thing they need to focus on is stress management. One client went so far to as say, "Danielle, it's not the food!" This woman was seeing how intertwined the rest of her life was with her eating habits and her health.

Could this be true for you too? How does stress show up in your life? Where are you feeling stretched beyond your limits? Where are you feeling pressure to be everything to everyone? Where are you working your guts out and excusing away your needs and wants? These are hard questions to ask, and it's even harder to start choosing differently, but that's what this chapter is about. Once you can get clear on what is stressing you out and what you can do about it, everything else will get easier. Stress management is absolutely crucial to vibrant living.

Stress management can take many different forms and have many different names. Another way to look at stress management is to call it "life balance." It's how you spend your time and energy. Stress management can be phrased more positively by calling it "self-care." Self-care is usually what's lacking in someone living with chronic stress. You can also think of it as energy management, time management, or even emotional wellness. All these count as stress management, and I may use these terms interchangeably. I hope you'll choose the one that is most meaningful to you.

What is stress, anyway? Well, your brain has two neural pathways: the sympathetic nervous system and the parasympathetic nervous system. When you are stressed, overwhelmed, frazzled, harried, and overworked, your sympathetic nervous system (SNS) runs the show. This is known as the "fight, flight, or freeze" response. When you are calm, at ease, settled, and peaceful, your body is working from the parasympathetic nervous system (PNS). This is the "rest and digest" mode. It's normal and natural to fluctuate between these two neurological responses throughout the day and throughout life. What is not healthful, though, is when you are constantly or chronically in fight-or-flight mode without recovering and returning to rest and digest mode.[18] Living this way is basically like pulling the fire alarm all day long. Nobody should have to live that way.

A comprehensive look at stress management is not possible in just one chapter. There are volumes written on this one subject alone. My intention in this chapter is to help you get clear and honest about how stress is showing up in your life and to give you some simple, practical next steps to improve your life balance, emotional wellness, self-care, etc. Are you ready to be honest with yourself about this? It's time to face the fact that you have needs and limits. You are not superhuman, and that's okay. Let me help you design a life that supports you rather than depletes you. Let's begin.

Stress: It's Mental and Physical

Stress is a big deal in modern life. If we lived more simply, it would not be as much of an issue. But here in the modern world, we live with lots of responsibilities, expectations, and a fast-paced environment we often struggle to keep up with. The stress this causes was never intended to be chronic. Biologically, stress was intended to help us give a jolt of adrenaline so we could flee immediate danger. But now, immediate danger comes in many forms that are much more mental than physical. Your stress will affect your physical and mental health. The Mayo Clinic identifies these common health risks of chronic stress:

- Anxiety
- Depression
- Digestive problems
- Headaches
- Heart disease
- Sleep problems
- Weight gain
- Memory and concentration impairment[19]

In modern life, these physical, mental, and emotional reactions to stress are your body trying to get your attention. What message is your body sending you? Are you listening? Or are you pushing it aside and ignoring the signals?

To tap into your motivation for facing stress and making changes to better manage it, be sure to go through the journal prompts at the end of this chapter. Where your stress comes from and how it manifests itself will be unique to you. How would stressing less help you start living the life you want?

When you are stressed, it's like making withdrawals on your energy bank account. If you want to continue to make withdrawals, you need to make consistent deposits. Where could you do more to make energy deposits? Think self-care and life balance here. Where are you not giving yourself the time and space to rest and recover?

Most givers and doers have a hard time slowing down enough to let this R & R happen. I know—I'm a recovering overachiever myself. I used to think the only thing worth doing was something that created results or helped others. I was chronically "productive." Can you relate? Do you feel like it's a waste when you sit for a moment to just be? Do you feel selfish when you take time for yourself? When you sit to read a book just for fun, does your mind race over your to-do list or "could-be-doing" list? If so, I give you permission to start loosening your grip on constantly doing and giving. After all, how can you keep giving and doing if you never pause to reset and recharge?

In this chapter, I'm going to give you some principles of stress management along with a few examples and suggestions for applying those principles in your daily life. This will only help you if you focus on your own life and think about how you can apply these principles in your own way. This will also require you to accept the idea that you can give and do more if you stress less. Commit now to finding ways to refill your cup so you can continue to give of yourself the way you want to.

Minimize, Recover, Maintain

What does it take to "manage" stress? Let me share an analogy I learned in my health-and-wellness coaching classes. One of my teachers specialized in stress, and she shared something called the "pond analogy." Picture a pond full of water. The pond is you, and the water is your capacity to handle the stressors in your life. Then let's say people start walking by all day long throwing rocks, pebbles, and an occasional boulder into your pond. You can imagine that with each offense, water splashes out and your capacity is compromised as your pond fills up with these stones and things. Does this sound a little like real life? I know it did for me when I first heard it. If you had a pond like this, what would you do to manage the situation? Go through this chapter's journal prompts to explore this further.

There are three things that need to happen to protect that pond: 1) you would need to minimize the number of stones that make it into the pond, 2) you would need to recover from the stressor by fishing the stones out and refilling the pond after each offense, and 3) you would need to make these protective and restorative measures a regular maintenance routine.

Can you see how our stress management is no different? One of the first things I focus on with clients who need to improve their stress management is boundaries. How much less would our "pond" be assaulted with stones and pebbles if we put up some good fences? A lot, right? Now, we probably don't want concrete walls, but maybe a nice picket fence with a gate to let those we care about in and out of our space. Boundaries can be permeable. We can establish healthy, reasonable boundaries that help us minimize stressors. Think about your own stressful situations. Where could saying no or having other boundaries support you in feeling better?

Recovering from stress is a huge part of healthy stress management. Most of us have ways we respond to stress, but they may not be very healthful ones. Emotional eating, anyone? Stress eating? These are the most common strategies, but they're not helpful. This is the next thing I focus on with clients, and it all comes back to the parts of a habit we talked about in chapter 6. When my boss gives me a huge assignment (trigger), I open my drawer and pull out a Ho-Ho from my sugar stash (behavior) so I can escape this feeling of overwhelm and have a glimmer of happiness from the sugar rush (payoff). Fill in the trigger, behavior, and payoff for your most stressful moments. What's triggering you? What's your go-to coping mechanism? What are you actually craving at that moment? The solution to breaking this cycle is this: What can you do instead to get that same payoff? Once you find what that is and create a new habit around it, you've created a healthy coping mechanism.

The final task is to have a regular maintenance routine that keeps you in tip-top shape. This is where self-care comes in. Only if you have regular routines that recharge, refill, and restore you are you staying ahead of the game. Only then will you increase your capacity for the ups and downs of life. Few of us do this naturally. We tend to face our stress management/energy management/life balance only when we hit rock bottom and can't take it anymore. What if you were proactive rather than reactive about your self-care? Commit to no longer running on empty. You wouldn't NOT fill your gas tank before going on a long trip, so why would you do that with your energy? It's time to take your self-care more seriously. Let's dive into what this can look like for you.

The Tools in Your Toolbox

If you had asked me a few years ago what I did for self-care, I would have had nothing to say. My idea of stress management was primarily having outlets to blow off steam, like running and weight lifting. I never slowed down. I never rested. I never stopped. But life eventually forced me to face my need to slow down. (Thank you again, car accident injury) I have learned the importance of rounding out my stress-management/self-care routine. I have worked hard to be able to answer four questions that I now extend to you.

What recharges you?

What do you do for fun?

How do you relax?

What makes you laugh out loud?

As you reflect, brainstorm, and experiment with the answers to these questions, you will be doing the most important work of self-care and stress management. Your answers will become the tools you can turn to as often as you need to be the balanced, happy person you most want to be.

I hired my own health-and-wellness coach to help me strengthen my self-care and stress-management repertoire, and I'm so glad I did. I'm a recovering overachiever, giver, and doer. I always had a hard time giving myself permission to take time for me. Speaking of which, let's talk more about time.

If you are a victim of your schedule, self-care and stress management will be almost impossible. When you guard your time, you protect your energy. For me, it was McKeown's message in his book *Essentialism* [20]that taught me to be daring and intentional about what I choose to say yes to and what I say no to. Essentialism (TM) is a way of living that invites you to let go of the nonessential things in an effort to bring forward your "highest possible contribution." The fact of the matter is that we will do more good when we do less of the non-essential things in our lives. Finding the "more in less" is a leap of faith, one I am glad I have taken. Are you struggling with balancing your life? Where are you over-extending yourself for others to the detriment of your own health and well-being? Spend time with the Journal Prompts at the end of this chapter to clarify this for yourself.

Let's go back to this idea of having an outlet. I have one. Actually, I have many. Mine are running, calling my mother, journaling, going for a walk, drumming on my drum set to my favorite music, and having a dance party for one in my kitchen. These things involve moving my body, being alone with my thoughts, or doing something that is plain fun, just for the heck of it. These things move me away from overthinking, stressing, worrying, and obsessing over the events of the day. Everyone needs an outlet. Even you. So what is it for you? Again, it will take some reflection, brainstorming, and experimenting on your part. That is the work of self-care and stress management. The things I just listed are the result of my own work in this area.

Let me suggest one practice that can help you if you need more than just an outlet or a little fun. If you struggle with any level of depression or anxiety, this one's for you.

Do you ever feel like your thoughts are running away without you? Mindfulness is the key to getting your brain back in your body. If you are a worrier, an overthinker, or just have a habit of staying stressed out all the time, mindfulness can help. Mindfulness is any practice that helps you feel more grounded and present in your physical body and less scattered and frenzied in your mental-emotional state. To me, mindfulness usually involves focusing on something physical in an effort to calm and distract myself from the mental and tune in to the emotional. Some of my favorite mindfulness practices are slow, deep breathing; tapping (or EFT); hiking; and cross-country skiing. **I have a few videos on things you might enjoy if you need more ways to practice mindfulness. Go to danielledinkelman.com/toolkit to view the bonus videos for this chapter**. My number-one suggestion: practice deep breathing every day. It's the quickest way to get grounded.

I hope I've struck a chord or two with you and sparked some ideas of things you can incorporate in your self-care/stress-management repertoire. If you take these ideas and turn them into routines, habits, rituals, and regular practices, you will get the most benefit out of them. Little habits make a big difference in managing time and energy. If it feels overwhelming to create habits around this, it's okay. We'll take it a step at a time.

Baby Steps to More Self-Care

Once you've begun to give yourself permission to take time for YOU, it's time to act.

If you're ready to make some changes, then find something, even something small, to start doing right now. Stake your claim. Drive your flag into the ground and say, "I am taking care of myself!" Commit and follow through. I get a little fired up about this because I have had so many clients who want to make changes in this area, but it takes a lot of talking and repeating and rehashing the new beliefs that give them permission to take time to take care of themselves. If you need to do that, then do it. Read this chapter on a daily basis if you have to!

That being said, I am a big fan of baby steps. If your sights are set on living a life where you take care of yourself, it's okay to work toward it one step at a time. Build self-care into your life one layer at a time.

My number-one tip in finding stress-management and self-care routines is the same for any other aspect of health and wellness. Stop looking for THE answer and start looking for YOUR answer. It's absolutely crucial your self-care routine is meaningful to YOU. Take my drum set, for example. My drumming outlet is incredibly cathartic and enormously fun for me! It's not something many other people would choose, but it's meaningful to me. I have wanted to play the drums since I was a kid, so it lights me up to have it in my life now. What about you? What would be cathartic for you? Spend time with this concept and find something that makes you feel like a kid in a candy store. We're looking for pure, geeky joy here.

Once you've got your sights set, make space in your life to do three things that fill your cup on a daily basis. These can be simple habits and routines. For me, it's 1) waking up before my kids do so I can study scriptures in peace, 2) taking a catnap most days after lunch, and 3) playing the drums while my kids are getting themselves a snack after school. These are the little things I do to demonstrate to myself (and my kids) that I am my own person with limits and needs. I make myself a priority. It's for my own good, and it's for their benefit too.

Self-Care Is Not Selfish

Remember—your stress will affect EVERYTHING. All aspects of your health and wellness are impacted by how well you practice stress management and self-care. When you take care of yourself, you are inherently taking care of others. My kids are like sponges and mirrors all wrapped into one. They soak up and reflect my mood and energy. The saying "If Momma ain't happy, ain't nobody happy" is all too true in my house. What about you? Have you noticed your stress or anxiety rubbing off on your loved ones? Your kids? What about at work? Does your stress affect the people you work with?

I believe that as you take care of yourself, everyone will thank you. Self-care is NOT selfish. It's taking care of yourself so you can be your highest self and be able to take better care of others.

What I hope you are taking from this chapter is a commitment to get ahead of your stress rather than be a victim of it. It's the difference between filling your car with gas on a regular basis instead of filling up only when the gas light turns on and you're running on fumes. It's a lot easier to stay ahead of self-care than it is to recover from crashing and burning.

I hope you are committing to the habit of managing your energy. I hope you are seeing how time management plays into self-care. I hope you see clearly how you can balance your life to make your mental and physical wellness a priority.

I talk to people every week that need to give themselves permission to put their health and wellness first. I hear story after story of women, and some men too, taking care of everyone else to the point they were dead last on their to-do lists. Women tend to define and then deplete themselves in the home. Men often do it with their careers. I've seen it go both! As I gently point this out, they agree that nothing will get better with nutrition or exercise or sleep until they decide to rearrange their lives to prioritize their self-care. It's time for a change.

Maybe this is your story too. If it is, aren't you tired of constantly reacting? Wouldn't it be nice to get ahead of things and be more proactive? I'll be the first to tell you, it's pretty heavenly. Stress management. Life balance. Self-care. Energy management. Emotional wellness. Mental health. Whatever you want to call it, it matters. Whatever you want to call it, YOU are in the driver's seat. I hope you will take this to heart and take those baby steps to living your life by design rather than by default.

Repeat after me:

- I am balanced.
- I am well.
- I am worth taking time to care for myself.
- I am making time for my self-care so I can be at my best and bless others better

TOOLKIT:

- YouTube Playlist - Mindfulness & Deep Breathing Video Playlist

CHAPTER 10 JOURNAL PROMPTS

1. How have you seen stress impact your day-to-day life? How is it impacting your health and wellness? How is your stress affecting the people around you?

2. Think of the pond analogy. How big is your pond? How full or shallow? How protected is it? Do you have a steady stream of self-care coming in to refill it? Or is it more like a trickle? Whatever the current state of your pond, know that you can take small steps to improve it.

3. What habits or practices do you want to adopt to feel less stressed and more balanced?

4. What small but mighty thing could you start doing to show yourself that you are prioritizing your self-care?

5. List at least twenty ways the OTHER PEOPLE in your life will benefit from you increasing your self-care and improving your stress management. Remind yourself of this often.

11

Sooner or Later, You'll Have to Face This

FROM THE VERY FIRST CLIENT I worked with, I knew there was one piece of the puzzle that affected nearly everyone. Mindset plays a huge role in how quickly and easily you will be able to make healthy changes. About six years ago, my eyes were opened to the power of mindset in my own life. The fact of the matter is that thoughts turn into feelings, feelings inform actions, and actions create results. Our thoughts (usually) begin with looking at our past experiences (or "results") and letting those shape how we see the world. These "thoughts" can become deeply ingrained beliefs about what is true in life. In fact, there's a whole canon of books written around the idea of "limiting beliefs."

When I started exploring my limiting beliefs, my life changed dramatically. Whether this idea is new to you or not, in this chapter, I will show you what limiting beliefs may stand in your way for creating a healthier lifestyle and how you can begin to shift into a new frame of mind. Whether you address this at the beginning of your journey, at the end, or throughout, that's fine. One way or another, if you want a new life, you'll need a new mindset.

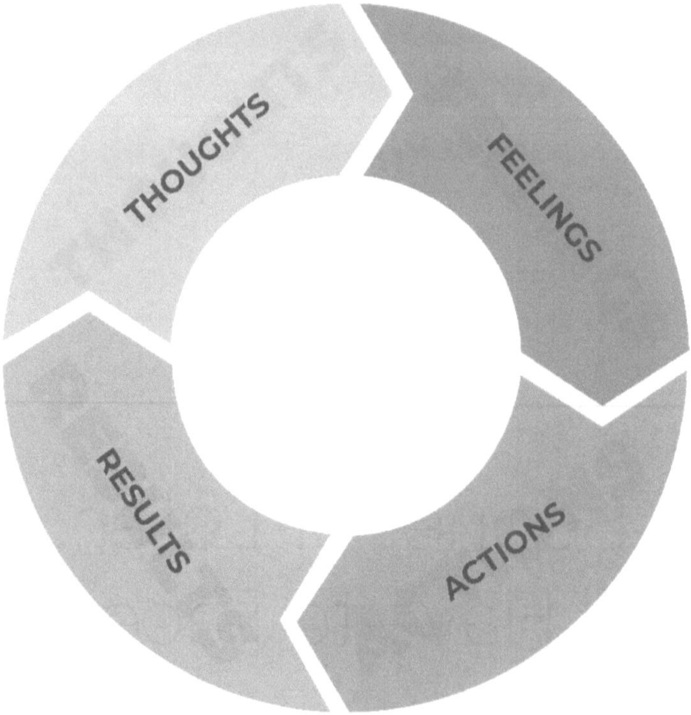

Henry Ford had it right when he said, "Whether you believe you can or can't, you're right." Some people might see limiting beliefs and mindset work as a little "out there." But the way I see it, it's just psychology. Remember the theory of self-efficacy—the idea that what we think we can or cannot do actually does impact whether we do it or not. Our thoughts matter. Sooner or later, you will have to face your thoughts, your beliefs, and your mindsets.

So the very first belief, or thought, I would like to bring to your attention is this: choose to believe this is possible for you. Thriving, living vibrantly again, changing your habits, reclaiming your health—it's all possible. Choose that thought for now. It might be hard to do, but it's okay to start small. I'll help you through some of the most important mindset shifts you'll need to be successful.

Your Thoughts Are Powerful

Have you discovered just how powerful your thoughts are? Even just the simple difference between positive thinking and negative thinking has been shown to have a huge impact on physical health.[21]

The long and short of it is that negative self-talk fuels stress, while positive self-talk diffuses it. Here are some known health benefits of positive thinking:

- Increased life span
- Lower rates of depression
- Lower levels of distress
- Greater resistance to the common cold
- Better psychological and physical well-being
- Better cardiovascular health and reduced risk of death from cardiovascular disease
- Better coping skills during hardships and times of stress

I know when I started focusing on the positive, my life experience changed completely. I was no longer just along for the ride and a victim of my circumstances. I started reframing negative things and letting them roll off my back rather than taking offense and letting them fester in my mind. Have you ever met a person that all they ever do is complain about how hard their life is? Compare that with the person who tries to see life on the bright side. Who is happier? Who do you enjoy being around more? Of course, positive thinking is not about ignoring the hard things in life and pretending to be okay no matter what. It's simply the practice of thinking differently in good and bad situations.

If positive thoughts were flowers and negative thoughts were weeds, which ones are you planting more of? Your thoughts are the seeds of your future. So why not start to be more intentional about the thoughts you choose?

In addition to the theory of self-efficacy, there's another behavior theory that focuses on the power of our thoughts and beliefs. Carol Dweck is a researcher whose work has uncovered the importance of a "growth mindset" and the detrimental effects of a "fixed mindset." Her TedTalk entitled, "The Power of Believing You Can Improve"[22] gives you a taste of what this is all about. These principles are being taught more and more in our schools, and they can help you on your health journey. My kids came home from school one day with a handout that said, "The power of yet" across the top. When you choose a growth mindset, you choose to believe you can improve. You say things like "I am not good at that YET." In one school I visited, there was a big poster with half listing the qualities of a growth mindset, the other half listing the qualities of a fixed mindset. It looked a little something like this:

"Failure is the limit of my abilities"
"I'm either good at it or I'm not"
"My abilities are unchanging"
"I don't like to be challenged"
"I can either do it or I can't"
"My potential is predetermined"
"When I'm frustrated, I give up"
"Feedback and criticism are personal"
"I stick to what I know"

"Failure is an opportunity to grow"
"I can learn to do anything I want"
"Challenges help me to grow"
"My effort and attitude determine my abilities"
"Feedback is constructive"
"I am inspired by the success of others"
"I like to try new things"

Which of these thoughts have you had around being able to turn your health around for good? Most of us have a little bit of both, of course, but do you see how powerful it could be to choose thoughts that cultivate a growth mindset? Do you see how limiting the thoughts of a fixed mindset can be? It's pretty striking when you see them side by side. "Limiting beliefs" is a thing. Here we have a psychological model for understanding limiting beliefs. So let's be aware of them, and let's reframe them.

It may be a little overwhelming or even defeating to know your thoughts have been shaping your reality. You might be tempted to beat yourself up about this. I have had clients feel that way. Heck, I sometimes feel that way! The biggest place I saw my thoughts and limiting beliefs show up was in my parenting. Once I learned about the power of my thoughts, I recognized that the "difficult" children I was raising might feel and act differently if MY thoughts, feelings, and actions were more intentional. You know what? I was right. As I

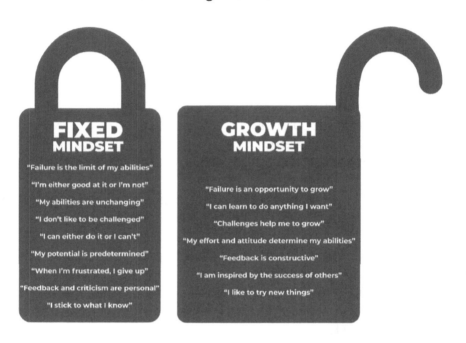

worked on my own "attitude adjustment," the dynamic in my relationship with my little ones completely changed. So the good news is that if we helped create our circumstances before, we can do it again. Once you pull back the curtain and know what thought processes are running in the background, you'll be able to do something about it. Once you see it, you can change it. Let's talk more about the thoughts and beliefs that may have been running the show with your health and wellness journey up to this point.

It's Time to Own Your Mindset

So, what are the mindsets you need to be aware of, and how can you change them? Let's first focus on the mindsets that may be undermining your best efforts to live a healthy lifestyle.

You can't change what you can't see. Once you see the mindsets, thoughts, and limiting beliefs for what they are, just knowing they are there will help you begin to shift them in a new direction.

Let's start with the victim mentality. If your life were a fairy tale or comic book, would you be the hero or the victim? Are you the one learning and growing and changing? Or are you the one crap always happens to and you're left crying for help? How do you see yourself? Which one do you WANT to be? Can you think of a few instances where you've been the hero? How about when you've been the victim? Circumstance does not determine which character you are, your thoughts do. Your perspective is what matters most. Are you simply letting life happen to you, or are you taking experiences and doing something constructive with them? Think of your favorite superhero movie. Hard stuff happens to the hero just as often as the poor unsuspecting victim. The difference is what they do with it.

All right, let's step back into the real world now. In addition to the victim mentality, there is another mindset I want you to be acquainted with. This one is more pervasive and harder to spot. It's camouflaged by societal norms. You see, some mindsets are cultural. You've been swimming in it, breathing in it, all your life. I'm talking about diet culture. If you've grown up in the United States, chances are your frame of reference for health and behavior change is influenced by diet culture. Remember chapter 2 and all the things that are wrong about diets? That's likely a big mindset shift you'll need to make. A few of the hallmark mindsets of diet culture are:

- No pain no gain.
- Big effort brings big reward.
- I'll be happy when I'm thin.
- If I'm not perfect, I won't be successful.
- I'll do whatever it takes to get my results.

As I shared in chapter 2, these do not serve you in a lifestyle approach to health and wellness. The lifestyle approach focuses on building habits, not white-knuckling our willpower. The lifestyle approach focuses on going slow and steady, not sprinting to the finish. The lifestyle approach focuses on sustainable progress over time rather than perfection now. The lifestyle approach focuses on gaining health rather than losing weight. This could be the most important mindset shift you make. Let go of diet culture and embrace a lifestyle mindset.

I believe it was Einstein who said, "You cannot solve a problem with the same thinking that created it." Wherever you are now with your mindset, you can take small steps out of the old and into the new. Whether you have been the hero or the victim, whether you have been thinking "diet" or lifestyle, mindsets are moldable. Be patient with yourself. You'll revert. It will be like closing a door behind you but once in a while turning around and bumping your head against it. You'll get to remind yourself, "Nope, I'm not doing it that way anymore." Thoughts, beliefs, and mindsets are just like any other habit, so let's look at how to start changing them.

Habits for a New Way of Thinking

Have you ever been stuck in your home for so long that just looking at the same four walls day after day after day made you want to redecorate? This is what happened to me when the COVID-19 pandemic hit. All of a sudden, I wasn't overly distracted with things outside my home. Just being inside more caused me to see what improvements needed to be made. It also gave me a lot of time to imagine what I would like things to look like. Remodeling your mindset is very much like remodeling your home—you have to spend time seeing it before you're ready to change it.

Now that you're aware of the power of your thoughts, there is plenty you can do to make some permanent upgrades. If noticing and changing your thoughts seems difficult at the moment, I have a trick for you. You can use your word choice to start shifting your mindset. Be mindful of how you talk to others about your life. Is it reflecting a victim mentality? When you're about to wallow in negativity, how can you adjust your word choice to reframe the negative into positive?

Some of the most powerful words we have are "I am." Everything that follows sends a message to your psyche and the rest of creation that this is who you are and this is how it is. Be careful of using the words "I am" in a fixed-mindset sort of way. Get out of the habit of saying things negatively or limiting yourself with those two very powerful words. Catch yourself when you are about to say things like, "I am just not good at this." Use "I am" carefully—like it's written in permanent ink. Use it to support your emerging growth mindset: "I am making progress." "I am practicing being patient." "I am learning so much."

Another way you can use your words to build your growth mindset and let go of a fixed mindset is to talk more about the process than the outcome: "I'm giving it my best." "I'm not there YET, but I will be one day." I do this with my kids in school when I say, "Wow, honey, you were so focused on your homework today" rather than "You did a good job; you got every math problem right!" See the difference? When we praise the process more than the outcome in ourselves and others, we allow space for growth and celebrate the thing that matters most.

If you're struggling with negative self-talk or a victim mentality, here is one mindset you can cultivate that will make all the difference: gratitude. Positivity starts with gratitude. When I first learned about the power of my thoughts, I began practicing gratitude in all my quiet moments. As I drove the kids to school, I would mentally list all the things I could be grateful for in that moment. The more I did this in the car, on walks, doing the dishes, and folding laundry, the more I cultivated an "attitude of gratitude." Now it's a part of who I am. I am always looking at the glass half full because it's a *habit* now. Repetition, repetition, repetition.

The power of our thoughts gives us permission and motivation to stop complaining and start creating. Our perspective actually shapes and creates our reality. Remember: thoughts lead to feelings, which inform actions, which create results in life. If you want a different life, you can start with creating a habit with how you use your thoughts and words.

Choose Your Thoughts, Change Your Life

I love working with clients who are willing to work on their mindset. It makes the process of change so much easier. It's the difference between snowshoeing and skiing. Both will get you to where you wanna go, but one is just so much more fun than the other! So how do you get there? How do you step into being the person who is willing to remodel your mindset to support this new life you want? Let's talk strategy.

First of all, please, please, please do not let this overwhelm you. Like everything else we've covered in this book, it's okay to take this a step at a time. You can pick one belief you want to shift. Which one of the suggestions in the last section resonated with you most? Gratitude? I am? Process over outcome? Any of these would make a HUGE difference in your mindset. So pick one and get to work. And remember, we're working smarter, not harder, when it comes to changing habits. So how can you use all three support systems to change your thought processes and word choices? Personally, socially, and environmentally, what can you do?

Amp up your personal ability and motivation to shift to more a empowered mindset by strengthening your understanding of the power of your thoughts. My favorite way to do this is to read! **I have put together a mindset book list and video about each one so you can choose what's best for you. These books have literally changed my life, and I know they can do the same for you. Go to danielledinkelman.com/toolkit to download the book list and watch the video that goes with it to hear my summary of each.** One of my favorite ways to make personal change more possible is to work with a therapist or counselor. I've worked with one over the years whenever things got dark or too difficult to handle on my own. I've had coaching clients who were in therapy while they worked on their health and wellness goals with me. I've gotta tell you—wellness coaching AND therapy is a powerful combination. If you could use some help sorting through your thoughts and feelings about the past and present, a therapist or counselor can really help. Don't be afraid of counseling. We ALL need a therapist sooner or later!

What about socially? How can you support a positive change in your thoughts and words in your social sphere? One way is to tell the people closest to you what you are working on. If you're working on gratitude or simple positive reframing, tell others about your intentions! Tell them about what you've learned and why you want to take control of your thoughts more. They'll help you catch yourself when you revert to old patterns. My mom and my husband did this for me, and you know what? They even came along on the journey! Now the two people I talk to most on this planet are in on it, too, and we are each intentional in thinking and speaking positively.

Environmentally is a little more elusive when it comes to mindset work. What could you add to or take out of your environment that will help you shift to a positive mindset? You could add music and media that is uplifting. You could add post-its and reminders that say, "I am . . ." or "Grateful" on them. You could opt out of TV shows and music that bring you down. What else in your physical surroundings would allow you and motivate you to think in the new way you want to? Paying attention to all three support systems will help you work smarter, not harder.

As you put these personal, social, and environmental supports in place to shift your mindset, take time to count your wins along the way. Celebrate the moments where you chose a different way of thinking. The more you recognize those moments, the more you will have them. Your momentum will build, the habit will emerge, and, soon enough, you'll have a totally new perspective that serves and supports you in building the life you want.

A New Mindset Will Bring Lasting Change

As I guide clients through lifestyle changes, the ones who stick with it are those who are thinking differently. The ones who keep reverting to old ways of doing are stuck in old ways of thinking. Remember, before action come feelings, and before feelings come thoughts. I'm so glad you've taken the time to read this chapter. Simply opening your eyes to the role mindset plays is a huge step forward. The work is already starting just with your new awareness.

As you practice some new thought habits, you might have moments like a client of mine once had. She called me up and shared a story about how she didn't react with the thoughts or feelings that usually came in a certain situation. She said, "Who is this person?" I told her, "It's the new you!" Trust and embrace the new you that will come as you shift your mindset. Soon enough, you'll be thinking and feeling in a whole new way about yourself, your life, and your health journey.

Now, what if you're feeling overwhelmed by the thought of tackling mindset head-on? That's okay. Do something small; even just starting with awareness is something. Again, counseling or therapy can be really powerful here if it's feeling too heavy to lift alone. But it's also okay to take a backdoor approach to mindset work. The way I do this with clients is to help them set achievable goals around other areas of their health, like nutrition or exercise. Then my job is to teach them to see the positive, focus on wins, and give themselves credit for the process more than the outcome. Bit by bit, week after week, their attitude begins to change and they get into the habit of looking on the bright side. It's a marvelous thing to see. If you could use this kind of support, go to danielledinkelman.com to learn more about working with me one-on-one or in our group coaching program.

Sooner or later, head-on, or backdoor approach, a new mindset will give you the life you want. This will unfold perfectly for you as long as you can be open to a new attitude. Choose to be open to new ways of thinking so you can fully and sustainably step into the new you and the vibrant life you want to be living.

TOOLKIT:

- Video + PDF - Mindset Book List

CHAPTER 11 JOURNAL PROMPTS

1. How much do you believe your thoughts, feelings, and attitudes impact your health and wellness? How much do your thoughts, feelings, and attitudes affect your ability to change?

2. What mindset do you see in yourself that has held you back?

3. What thinking and speaking habits would help you remodel your mindset and attitudes about life, yourself, and getting healthy?

4. Where will you begin? What's your first baby step in remodeling your mindset?

5. How will thinking differently about yourself, your life, and your health and wellness help you be successful in creating the life you want?

12

Feel Your Best So You Can Give Your All

YOU DID IT! YOU MADE IT all the way to the end. I am so proud of you for taking the time to learn a new and better way to reclaim your health with a lifestyle approach. You know, the fact that you kept reading all the way to the end and stayed with me through the uncomfortable parts is pretty exceptional because only 30 percent of readers tend to finish the books they start. Go ahead and pat yourself on the back for following through on this commitment. You finished what you started!

I want you to know that I believe in lifestyle medicine. You know, even the World Health Organization believes in lifestyle medicine! Their numbers show that about 80 percent of chronic diseases, like heart disease, stroke, diabetes, and even cancer, are lifestyle-related.[23] In fact, in some circles, these diseases are referred to as "lifestyle diseases."

Our day-to-day habits and behaviors either work for us or against us. Over and over, I have seen clients who choose the path I've laid out for you in this book and truly start to feel better. I believe that feeling better is a lot simpler than most of us think. You have everything you need to start feeling better now. You now know WHAT to focus on, HOW to go about changing your habits, and WHY you want to keep working on them.

You deserve to feel better. You deserve to take the time, energy, and money you need to care for yourself so you can feel better. So many people depend on you and care about you. They want you to feel better. If you have been living with chronic fatigue, depression, anxiety, or any sort of lifestyle disease, I hope you now have a spark of hope within you. I hope you feel you have a say in what comes next.

A client who recently started working with me had already improved her diet to almost all wholesome, natural foods (aka whole-food, plant-based), so she wasn't sure if she needed much help. As we talked more about her health and wellness, though, she told me she suffered from a constant, nagging anxiety. My visceral reaction was: *That is not okay*! My heart nearly leapt out of my chest for her. As we looked at other areas of wellness, sure enough, her nutrition was in good shape, but her sleep and stress management were in shambles, as was her exercise. I have high hopes for this client now that we are working to implement new habits. I am confident the work she is doing will help her feel better.

What about you? What have you been living with and accepting as your fate? Do you believe you can turn things around? I believe you can. Find your hope and don't let go.

Sometimes all you need is a little more clarity, focus, and momentum. That's what my clients get when they work with me, whether it's one-on-one or in my group coaching program. I love working with people who have woken up to the fact that they deserve to feel better and that better is possible for them. You can learn more about the work I do in my coaching practice in the bonus chapter that follows and at www.danielledinkelman.com. **In fact, by reading this entire book, you have earned a free forty-five-minute VIP coaching session with me! Send an email to hello@danielledinkelman.com and tell me how you're feeling after finishing this book. Send me the Journal Prompts you completed along the way, and I'll send you a scheduling link to set up your VIP coaching session. Use the subject line: "I finished what I started!" I want to hear from you.**

Now, as you finish this final chapter of our journey, let's pull it all together so you can see and feel how this lifestyle approach works to help you feel your best and give your all. Let's review what it will take for you to be successful.

Remember Your "Why"

It's a powerful thing to start with "why." Why do you want to feel better? Are you crystal clear on that yet? How will life be different as you start to feel better? If that is hard to answer, maybe you can answer a question that explores the flip side of that. Have you ever considered where your health and your life is headed if you do nothing? If you keep going the way you're going, what will happen? In life, in relationships, in health, in finances, or in happiness, where will you be if you don't choose another path? For some, it might mean crippling health problems. For others, it might mean mental and emotional despair and dysfunction. At the very least, you may see yourself on a path to unhappiness and unfulfilled potential.

This reality check may be sobering, but it's worth facing.

You know me well enough by now to know that I'm not a fan of focusing on the negative for too long. Let it do its eye-opening work and then turn your attention to all the positive reasons you have for choosing a new path. How about this: Who will you be influencing for the better as you turn your health around with your lifestyle? Who is watching you? How will *you* taking better care of *you* impact other people? Think of your friends, your family, your coworkers—anyone you are connected to.

I have worked with clients who deeply want to set a better example for the people in their life. One client wanted to influence their sister. Another wanted to show her children the way to live healthier. Of course, you first need to change for yourself, but it doesn't hurt to be mindful of the good you could be doing for others by taking care of yourself. For so many people, especially women and men who live in the service of others, it can feel selfish to take so much time, money, and energy for one's self in this lifestyle approach to health. But I've said it before, and I'll say it again: getting healthier could be the most selfless thing you ever do. I hope you can see that, feel that, and own that.

Now that you are crystal clear on your "why," let's review exactly what you'll need to do to take this new path to health and wellness. What does the lifestyle approach require?

You Can Live Vibrantly Now

In my mind, this lifestyle approach can start right now. Of course, it will take time to put new habits in place and begin to feel all the benefits you crave, but you can live vibrantly now. You can show up for yourself today by simply making a commitment to choose vibrant living. Even if it begins only in your mind and your attitude. Here's what I hope you would adopt in this new lifestyle of yours:

The new you makes health a priority. You take the time, money, and energy to care for yourself. You are aware of and working toward:

1. Prioritizing sleep
2. Improving nutrition
3. Enjoying regular exercise
4. Intentionally managing stress
5. Slowly but surely remodeling mindsets

You do not put all your eggs in one basket. You know the power of all five of these aspects of health and wellness.

The new you is patient. You are content in your progress. You start with what feels doable. You stay in your learning zone. You are mindful of balancing your ability with the challenge of new things so you can stay in your flow. You move onward and upward as you are self-aware enough to stay out of your panic zone. You keep moving forward.

You are committed to enjoying the journey. You know it will take effort and commitment, but you are here to create a healthy life-style you love and will love you back. You know yourself, your val-ues, your personality, and as such you know what your non-nego-tiables are as you create a new lifestyle for yourself. You lean into your strengths and find YOUR way of moving forward.

You know that each small change makes a big difference over time. You commit to moving forward, not backward. You see setbacks as opportunities to learn and adjust. You believe in the compound effect of small steps over time. You trust the process.

Speaking of the process, let's review the "how" of this lifestyle approach to health. It's the key to leaving dieting behind forever and leaning into a better way to change.

Find Your Rhythm

Going from the mainstream dieting world to an intentional lifestyle approach is no easy task. It's like hiking in a forest where there is no trail. You know the general direction you want to go, but it's easy to get disoriented when there's no clear path under your feet.

I am committed to helping each of my clients find and follow their own path. I get to be the guide who helps them navigate the underbrush and encourages them to keep moving forward.

Really, the biggest difference between a dieting approach and a lifestyle approach is that dieting works from the outside in and lifestyle changes work from the inside out. Lasting change comes from the inside out. You need to be in touch with who you are, how you move through life, and what is most important to you, then let that be your compass every step of the way. A good coach will draw that out of you.

But what if you're not working with a coach? How can you find your own path in all of this? Well, I'll tell you. There is a very simple cycle of thought that guides my coaching. I'll teach it to you now if you like. Or you can experience it for yourself in one of my coaching programs. If you know you're the type of person who would be more successful and consistent with a little hand-holding, you can learn about working with me in the bonus chapter that comes next.

Here's the simple rhythm I take all my coaching clients through: dream, plan, act, reflect, dream, plan, act, reflect. This is how we make unstoppable progress. This is what it takes to make a change from the inside out. Mindfully moving through each stage of this cycle will give you the self-awareness needed to follow your own path and never stop moving forward. I dive into this more deeply in my group coaching program, VIBRANT Living, but if you are hungry for more, **I'll walk you through each of these stages in the *Doing the Work* video found at danielledinkelman.com/toolkit.**

This process of becoming more self-aware will not only keep you moving forward but force you to practice tapping into your intuition, plan your next steps, mindfully act on your plan, and reflect on what worked and what didn't. Can you see and feel how transformative a process this is? Talk about changing from the inside out. As my clients get used to this rhythm and go through this cycle again and again, their confidence, self-trust, and intuition grow. I see it, and it brings me so much joy. It's the self-improvement and personal development that comes from this process that convinces me of the truth of the cryptic saying "The journey is the destination."

Self-awareness is the process, or the "how," of moving forward with the lifestyle approach. Bear in mind, though, whether you're doing this on your own or working with a coach, one way or another, you must carve out time to do this self-awareness work. Taking time to think is essential. That is where your lessons learned and next steps will be waiting for you. With a strong self-awareness, your success is inevitable as long as you just keep going.

Start Where You Are, Then Take the Next Step

So, where do you go from here? You've seen the whole picture. You've got all the pieces. How do you start putting this puzzle together for YOU? Well, here is where I'm going to remind you that slow and steady wins the race. This is where I will tell you again that you do not need to do this all at once. I hope you see a new way to make changes that does not require an iron will, a white-knuckle grip, or grinning and bearing it.

Here are your next steps: **Create your own Wellness Blueprint. In your toolkit, there's a walkthrough video and a blueprint work-**

book for you to design YOUR next steps for the first ninety days. You'll create your vision statement, choose two or three areas of focus, set ninety-day-habit goals, and identify the obvious action steps. Then it's up to you to take baby steps—small but mighty baby steps—to put your plan into action.

So go make your plan. You've got this! And I've got you. You can re-read this book as often as you need to. It will help you stay grounded in this new way of thinking about health and wellness. You can do this. Do the work. Show up for yourself. Know your "edge" and respect it. Remember to work smarter, not harder. Keep moving forward with self-awareness. Remember that "failure" is never final if you learn from it. Whatever comes, just keep going.

When I was embarking on something really big and important to me, I was reading a book called *Shoe Dog.*[24] It's the story of Nike, by founder Phil Knight. Phil was a long-distance runner and gritty entrepreneur, so he knew what it was like to tackle something big and important. This piece of advice he gives in the first few pages of his book applies beautifully to any worthy goal: "Keep going until you get there, and don't give much thought to where 'there' is." At first blush, you might think, "Wait, am I not supposed to keep my eye on the prize?" Yes and no. It's great to set your sights on where you're headed, but when it comes to the day-to-day, you've just gotta keep putting one foot in front of the other. In the work of turning your health around with lifestyle medicine, just focus on creating the habits and let your health and wellness take care of themselves. Because they will.

Love Is the Strongest Motivator

When things get hard, don't go back to the self-hatred diet culture teaches. Don't beat yourself up; it doesn't help.

The thing that separates the true lifestyle approach to health from diet tactics is self-compassion. You can give yourself some grace when things are not working the way you hoped. One of the most loving things you can say to yourself when you fall into old habits is, "I did the best I could at the time." The best thing you can do next is try, try again. Revisit the chapters in this book and look for answers on how you can set yourself up for success. Remember, this is not all up to you. Use the tools in this book to design support personally, socially, and environmentally.

I hope instead of punishing yourself into submission, you'll speak kindly to yourself. I hope you'll find a way to focus on health and wellness from a place of positivity, self-love, and self-care. I see choosing health as an act of love: Love for yourself. Love for an amazing body that keeps you breathing and moving every day. Love for the family and friends who depend on and care for you. Love of life and all the joy and adventure it has to offer. And then there's the love of God and his love for you. I believe in a God who is our father. I believe he gave us these amazing bodies as a gift to live and learn and have joy and to serve and do good. Whatever you believe, I hope you can see your body as a gift. I hope you can love yourself into good health so you can enjoy the bounties of a healthier, happier life.

The life you want can be yours. The process will be beautiful and expanding. The journey can be hard, but it's doable. Challenging, but enjoyable. It's not either/or. It's both/and. I hope you will watch and wonder at what unfolds for you. I believe you can do this. One step at a time, you can do this.

Now, before I leave you to it, I have one more thing to ask of you. If this book has resonated with you, if it has helped and encouraged you, will you please share it with someone who needs that help and encouragement? I believe we are on this planet to help one another, and I know you believe that too. The things you do, the things you say, and the books you share can be life-changing for those around you. So please pay it forward, and let's show the world there's a better way to live the life you want.

Take care, my friend. Take care and be well.

TOOLKIT:

- Doing the Work video
- Blueprint Walkthrough video
- Blueprint workbook

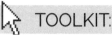

CHAPTER 12 JOURNAL PROMPTS

1. What is your "why"? Remember to go five layers deep if you can.

2. What areas of focus did you choose to start with? What are your three-month-habit goals in those areas? (For guidance on making your three -month plan, download the Wellness Blueprint Videos & Workbook.)

3. What routines around dreaming, planning, acting, and reflecting will you follow? Consider daily, weekly, monthly, quarterly, and yearly routines.

4. Where do you tend to push too hard in your health-and-wellness goals? What will you do to remind yourself to take it one step at a time?

5. When you feel like quitting, what will you do to bring yourself back? Who can help you make sure you find your flow and that you are giving yourself grace for your setbacks and credit for your accomplishments?

Getting the Support You Need

Leaving diet culture behind and being successful in a lifestyle approach to health can be challenging. If you are looking for support throughout your process, I am here for you. Coaching is available depending on your budget and your desired level of support. To learn more about group coaching and individual coaching with me, go to danielledinkelman.com

To reward you for your time and effort in reading this book and completing the journal prompts along the way, you now have access to a free 45 min VIP Coaching Session with me! Simply email your completed Journal Prompt Workbook to me at hello@danielledinkelman.com to request your free session. We'll discuss what you learned in the book and create a plan of action for your next steps.

I am here to support women and men in reclaiming their health with lifestyle. My group program currently is for women only, but I do work with men in my individual coaching practice. If you did not get a chance to complete the journal prompts and you simply want to learn more about which program would be a good fit for you, book a 20 min Discovery Call at danielledinkelman.com

Coaching is a powerful investment that can transform self-awareness, shift mindset, and create powerful habits for overall success and wellbeing. Growth does not happen overnight, which is why all of my coaching programs are a six month minimum commitment. Following are the details for my two coaching options. Feel free to contact me with any questions.

Individual Health & Wellness Coaching

In my **individual health & wellness coaching practice, I help women and men find and develop clarity, focus, and momentum in their health journey.** We focus on your personal goals and challenges and create a customized, doable, enjoyable plan to help you create the life you want.

Here's what it looks like:

- **Regular telephone coaching sessions (monthly, semi-monthly, or weekly sessions)** —discuss your successes and setbacks to examine lessons learned and plan small adjustments and next steps toward your wellness goals

- ***Wellness Blueprint Session* (90 min zoom session)—**personalized guidance in defining your vision, areas of focus, three-month goals, and action steps unique to you

- **3 Lifestyle Change Workshops—**learn the language of behavior change and how to take sustainable steps to make your journey more successful than ever before

    - *How to Life-Proof Your Goals*
    - *How to Take Charge of Your Habits*
    - *How to Support the Changes You Make*

- **Full access to VIBRANT Living (women only at this time) —**give and receive community support and learn from others working on similar goals as you

When you are overcoming deep-seated mindsets leftover from diet culture, your confidence in your ability to change may be down to zero. This is when a personal health coach can help the most to get you back on your feet and making progress in your journey. You do not have to do this alone.

To learn more and find out if coaching is right for you; request a free discovery call at danielledinkelman.com.

VIBRANT Living Group Coaching Program

In my **VIBRANT Living Coaching Program, I help women find and develop clarity, focus, and momentum in their health journey.** I want to help women who have struggled in the past to be successful, once and for all. (I do work with men, but only in my 1x1 coaching.)

In VIBRANT Living, we focus on bringing everything you read in this book to life. We help you apply it in a way that is personal and meaningful to you.

Here's what it looks like:

Two group coaching sessions per month—to share your successes and setbacks to keep learning and progressing toward your wellness goals

- ***Wellness Blueprint Walkthrough* video and workbook—** to guide you through defining your vision, three-month goals, and action steps to success

- **Private Facebook group—**so we can cheer each other on throughout the week, share recipes, and connect with others who are choosing the lifestyle approach to health and wellness

- **Ongoing trainings and workshops about all things Vibrant Living**—vision, values, habits, goals, support, sleep, nutrition, exercise, self-care, mindset, and more!

The biggest challenge in healthy living is sticking with it. Inside VIBRANT Living, we are committed to sustainable change and being mindful and intuitive along the way. Maintain your momentum. Keep your clarity. Join us inside.

To join, request a free discovery call at danielledinkelman.com.

I believe better is possible for you. You can do this!

Acknowledgments

THIS BOOK HAS BEEN FORMING IN my heart and mind for years. I am grateful for God's encouragement and guidance. Without it, I never could have written this book.

Thank you to my husband for never guffawing at my big ideas. Your love gives me the room to grow.

Thank you to my children—the four in my home and the one in my heart—who inspire me every day to show them what is possible. Thank you for cheering me on and letting me be both your mother and myself.

Thank you to my coaches. I could not have done this without you.

- Rebecca MacFarlane for believing in a brand-new coach and businesswoman
- Tara Newman for showing me how to lead boldly
- Elise Smith for keeping me grounded in God's purpose for my work
- Tiffany Berg Coughran for showing me how fun and rewarding it can be to write a book
- Yvette Morton for helping me prioritize my self-care and manage stress with love and wisdom
- Suzanna Cooper for opening my eyes to the big picture , and the life-changing magic of asking the right questions

Finally, thank you to my readers. I wrote this book for you because you deserve to feel ENJOY feeling healthy.

Launch Team Members

Georgia Davis
Rebecca Roberts
Tia Johansen
Tricia Schroeder
Chriti Pierson
Sandra Harrah
Katherine Van Alfen
Laurie Green
Jessica Clayson
Michelle Farrell
Christi Brinkmann
Mary Ann Garces
Maryellen Boyce
Angela Palmer
Ron Goral
Judy Shepherd
Julie Adams

Tawnya Fackrell
Dion Fowles
Cara O'Sullivan
Jocelyn Michael
Alexis Ford-Green
Misti Robinson
Mark Rasmussen
Emma Cowley
Adele Marcum
Jill Helsel
Janette Franson
DeOnna Braunberger
Stacy Milardovic
Dawn Brooks
Jubilee Rasmussen
Tepoerava Ka'aumoana
Karen Walley

Endnotes

1 Christina Weiss, "Statistics on Dieting and Eating Disorders," Monte Nido: Treating Eating Disorders, retrieved February 19, 2021,https://www.montenido.com/pdf/montenido_statistics.pdf.

2 Ibid.

3 Linda Searing, "The Big Number: 45 Million Americans Go on a Diet Each Year," *The Washington Post*, 2017 https://www.washingtonpost.com/national/health-science/the-big-number-45-million-americans-go-on-a-diet-each-year/2017/12/29/04089aec-ebdd-11e7-b698-91d4e35920a3_story.html.

4 "Wellness Is a Choice," The Wellspring, 2018, http://www.thewellspring.com/wellspring/introduction-to-wellness/357/key-concept-1-the-illnesswellness-continuum.cfm.html.

5 James O. and Janice M. Prochaska, Changing to Thrive: Using the Stages of Change to Overcome the Top Threats to Your Health and Happiness (Center City, Minnesota: Hazelden, 2016).

6 Marie Kondo, The Life Changing Magic of Tidying Up: The Japanese Art of Decluttering and Organizing (Berkeley, CA: Ten Speed Press, 2010).

7 Charles Duhigg, The Power of Habit: Why We Do What We Do in Life and Business (New York: Random House, 2012).

8 Wendy Wood, Good Habits, Bad Habits: The Science of Making Positive Changes That Stick (New York: Farrar, Straus, and Giroux, 2019).

9 Mihaly Csikszentmihalyi, *Flow: The Psychology of Optimal Experience* (New York: Harper & Row, 1990).

10 Center for Disease Control, "A Good Night's Sleep Is Critical for Good Health," CDC Newsroom, February 16, 2016, https://www.cdc.gov/media/releases/2016/p0215-enough-sleep.html.

11 Center for Disease Control, "Tips for Better Sleep," July 15 2016, CDC, https://www.cdc.gov/sleep/about_sleep/sleep_hygiene.html.

12 Center for Disease Control, "How Much Sleep Do I Need?" March 2 2017, https://www.cdc.gov/sleep/about_sleep/how_much_sleep.html.

13 Michael Klaper, Moving Medicine Forward, accessed February 19, 2021, https://www.doctorklaper.com/.

14 Caldwell B. Esselstyn, Jr., *Prevent & Reverse Heart Disease* (New York: Avery, 2007); *Dean Ornish's Program For Reversing Heart Disease* (New York: Ballantine Books, 1990).

15 Katherine D. McManus, "Should I Be Eating More Fiber?" Harvard Health Publishing, February 27, 2019, https://www.health.harvard.edu/blog/should-i-

be-eating-more-fiber-2019022115927.

16 World Health Organization, "Physical Inactivity a Leading Cause of Disease and Disability, Warns WHO" WHO Departmental News, April 4, 2002, https://www.who.int/news/item/04-04-2002-physical-inactivity-a-leading-cause-of-disease-and-disability-warns-who.

17 Department of Health and Human Services, "Top 10 Things to Know About the Second Edition of the Physical Activity Guidelines for Americans," Health.gov, October 7 2020, https://health.gov/our-work/physical-activity/current-guidelines/top-10-things-know.

18 Rachel Nall, reviewed by Seunggu Han, "Your Parasympathetic Nervous System Explained," April 23, 2020, https://www.healthline.com/health/parasympathetic-nervous-system.

19 Mayo Clinic Staff, "Chronic Stress Puts Your Health at Risk," Mayo Clinic, March 19, 2019, https://www.mayoclinic.org/healthy-lifestyle/stress-management/in-depth/stress/art-20046037.

20 Greg McKeown, Essentialism: The Disciplined Pursuit of Less (New York: Currency, 2014).

21 Mayo Clinic Staff, "Positive thinking: Stop Negative Self-Talk to Reduce Stress," Mayo Clinic, January 21, 2020, https://www.mayoclinic.org/healthy-lifestyle/stress-management/in-depth/positive-thinking/art-20043950.

22 Carol Dweck, "The Power of Believing That You Can Improve," Ted, January 21, 2020, https://www.ted.com/talks/carol_dweck_the_power_of_believing_that_you_can_improve/up-next?language=en.

23 Walter C. Willett, Jeffrey P. Koplan, Rachel Nugent, Courtenay Dusenbury, Pekka Puska, and Thomas A. Gaziano, "Prevention of Chronic Disease by Means of Diet and Lifestyle Changes," 2006, https://www.ncbi.nlm.nih.gov/books/NBK11795/.

24 Phil Knight, Shoe Dog: A Memoir by the Creator of NIKE (New York: Scribner, 2016).

Made in United States
Troutdale, OR
02/14/2024

17684375R00096